The Gym Workout
Body Sculpting

Fitness, Health & Nutrition was created by Rebus, Inc. and published by Time-Life Books.

REBUS, INC.

Publisher: RODNEY FRIEDMAN
Editorial Director: CHARLES L. MEE JR.

Editor: THOMAS DICKEY
Executive Editor: SUSAN BRONSON
Senior Editor: WILLIAM DUNNETT
Associate Editors: MARY CROWLEY, CARL LOWE
Copy Editor: LINDA EPSTEIN
Contributing Editor: JACQUELINE DAMIAN

Art Director: JUDITH HENRY
Associate Art Director: FRANCINE KASS
Designer: SARA BOWMAN
Photographer: STEVEN MAYS
Photo Stylist: LINDSAY DIMEO
Photo Assistant: TIMOTHY JEFFS

Test Kitchen Director: GRACE YOUNG
Recipe Editor: BONNIE J. SLOTNICK
Contributing Editor: MARYA DALRYMPLE
Chief of Research: CARNEY W. MIMMS III
Assistant Editor: PENELOPE CLARK

Time-Life Books Inc. is a wholly owned subsidiary of

TIME INCORPORATED

Founder: HENRY R. LUCE 1898-1967

Editor-in-Chief: JASON MCMANUS
Chairman and Chief Executive Officer: J. RICHARD MUNRO
President and Chief Operating Officer: N.J. NICHOLAS JR.
Corporate Editor: RAY CAVE
Executive Vice President, Books: KELSO F. SUTTON
Vice President, Books: GEORGE ARTANDI

TIME-LIFE BOOKS INC.

Editor: GEORGE CONSTABLE

Executive Editor: ELLEN PHILLIPS
Director of Design: LOUIS KLEIN
Director of Editorial Resources: PHYLLIS K. WISE
Editorial Board: RUSSELL B. ADAMS JR., DALE M. BROWN, ROBERTA CONLAN, THOMAS H. FLAHERTY, LEE HASSIG, DONIA ANN STEELE, ROSALIND STUBENBERG, KIT VAN TULLEKEN, HENRY WOODHEAD
Director of Photography and Research: JOHN CONRAD WEISER

President: CHRISTOPHER T. LINEN
Chief Operating Officer: JOHN M. FAHEY JR.
Senior Vice President: JAMES L. MERCER
Vice Presidents: STEPHEN L. BAIR, RALPH J. CUOMO, NEAL GOFF, STEPHEN L. GOLDSTEIN, JUANITA T. JAMES, HALLETT JOHNSON III, CAROL KAPLAN, SUSAN J. MARUYAMA, ROBERT H. SMITH, PAUL R. STEWART, JOSEPH J. WARD
Director of Production Services: ROBERT J. PASSANTINO

Editorial Operations
Copy Chief: DIANE ULLIUS
Production: CELIA BEATTIE
Library: LOUISE D. FORSTALL

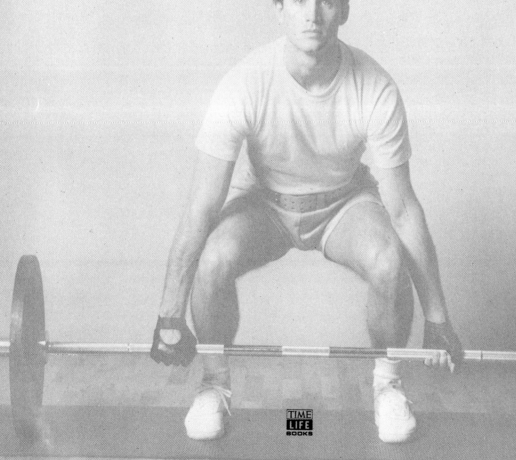

FITNESS, HEALTH & NUTRITION

The Gym Workout
Body Sculpting

TIME
LIFE
BOOKS

Time-Life Books, Alexandria, Virginia

CONSULTANTS FOR THIS BOOK

William D. McArdle, Ph.D., is a professor in the Department of Health and Physical Education at Queens College of the City University of New York. Dr. McArdle is a Fellow of the American College of Sports Medicine. Among his books are *Exercise Physiology: Energy, Nutrition, and Human Performance; Getting in Shape* and *Nutrition, Weight Control, and Exercise.*

Ann Grandjean, Ed.D., is Associate Director of the Swanson Center for Nutrition, Omaha, Neb.; chief nutrition consultant to the U.S. Olympic Committee; and an instructor in the Sports Medicine Program, Orthopedic Surgery Department, University of Nebraska Medical Center.

Myron Winick, M.D., is the R.R. Williams Professor of Nutrition, Professor of Pediatrics, Director of the Institute of Human Nutrition, and Director of the Center for Nutrition, Genetics and Human Development at Columbia University College of Physicians and Surgeons. He has served on the Food and Nutrition Board of the National Academy of Sciences and is the author of many books, including *Your Personalized Health Profile.*

The following consultants helped design the exercises in this book:

Ralph Anastasio has a master's degree in exercise physiology and physical education and is certified both as an exercise program director and an exercise test technologist by the American College of Sports Medicine. He is the general manager of an athletic club in New York City.

Michael A. Motta, the director of a fitness clinic in New York City, works as a personal athletic trainer. He holds a master's degree in physical education and has completed work leading to a Doctorate of Education in exercise physiology. In addition, Motta has taught physical education and served as a coach at the State University of New York at Albany.

Richard Weil is an exercise physiologist who has designed weight-training programs for a number of athletic clubs. He is a certified exercise test technologist. Weil has also been a member of the All-American Fencing Team.

For information about any Time-Life book please call 1-800-621-7026, or write:
Reader Information
Time-Life Customer Service
P.O. Box C-32068
Richmond, Virginia 23261-2068

First printing.
Published simultaneously in Canada.
School and library distribution by Silver Burdett Company, Morristown, New Jersey.

TIME-LIFE is a trademark of Time Incorporated U.S.A.

Library of Congress Cataloging-in-Publication Data
The Gym workout.
(Fitness, health & nutrition)
Includes index.
1. Weight training. I. Time-Life Books.
II. Series: Fitness, health, and nutrition.
GV546.G96   1988   646.7′5   88-2209
ISBN 0-8094-6106-4
ISBN 0-8094-6107-2 (lib. bdg.)

This book is not intended as a medical guide or a substitute for the advice of a physician. Readers are urged to consult a physician before beginning any program of strenuous physical exercise.

CONTENTS

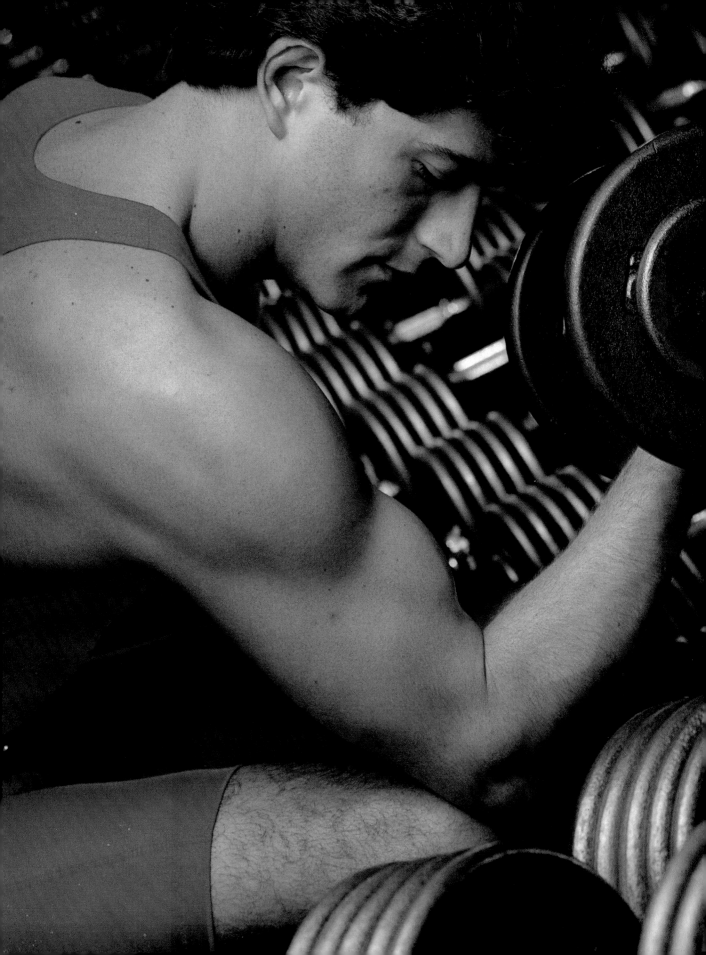

CHAPTER ONE

Working with Weights

Using progressive resistance to build a well-defined body

Once the domain of competitive body builders and weight lifters, weight training has gained far wider appeal in recent years among both men and women. Although lifting weights can produce dramatic increases in muscle bulk, for the average person the chief benefit is to enhance the shape and definition of muscles, along with providing a modest increase in muscle size. Perhaps more than any other type of exercise, weight training allows you to see the results of your effort: Working with weights is the quickest, most efficient way to sculpt specific muscles, as well as to improve the shape and tone of your overall physique. Other benefits include improved posture, better performance in other activities and better protection from injuries. But while weight training is an excellent way to develop and maintain a strong, well-shaped body, the variety of methods and regimens available is bewildering. This book will help you choose a program that suits your own goals.

What types of exercises and exercise equipment does weight training include?

Weight training involves using weight-loaded devices that you move in a variety of ways — lifting, pressing, pushing, pulling, curling — to work the body's various muscle groups. One way to perform such exercises is with free-weight equipment, which includes barbells — long bars with adjustable weights on each end — and dumbbells, shortened barbells that can be gripped with one hand. Free weights are the most commonly used type of weight-training equipment.

Weight training can also be performed with specially designed machines. Some of these have been used by body builders and athletes for decades — for example, Universal machines that have multiple stations for exercising all the major muscle groups. In the past 20 years, highly sophisticated machines have been designed to overload muscles with greater efficiency than free weights by utilizing such mechanisms as cams to move stacks of weights or hydraulic cylinders to provide resistance to movement. This equipment, which includes Nautilus machines, is both large and expensive, and for that reason it is found mainly in health clubs and other commercial gyms and training facilities.

With either free weights or machines, you can control the work load of an exercise by adjusting the amount of weight you lift. The key to building muscles is to start out by lifting a manageable amount of weight and, as you get stronger, increasing the amount — a process referred to as progressive resistance training. By adapting to this ever-increasing demand of weight loading, the muscles become stronger, larger and more defined.

Are there other methods of strengthening and shaping muscles?

Yes, but they are not as effective. For example, sit-ups, push-ups and the like will tone and firm muscles, but with these calisthenics, you are working against a fixed resistance — your own body weight. You can increase the demand on muscles in other ways, such as by performing an exercise more rapidly, so that you have less time to rest. But weight training allows you to overload your muscles systematically and with great precision, and for that reason it has been the cornerstone of the most effective strength-building regimens. In a study of Navy men, for example, a group that participated in a combination aerobics and weight-training program was compared with a second group that followed an aerobics and calisthenics program. After eight weeks, the weight-training group had made significant strength gains, while the second group had not.

What happens to a muscle when you train it with a progressive resistance regimen?

The body responds in a number of ways to the process of muscle overloading. First, it makes neurological adaptations, changes in the nervous system involving the way in which messages are passed from

Weight training may help decrease stress as it increases strength and muscle mass. In one experiment, strength-trained college athletes and untrained but physically active students performed series of squats — squatting and rising with a barbell resting on the shoulders. At any given weight load and intensity, the trained subjects showed lower heart rates, a reduced awareness of exertion and a faster heart rate recovery — adaptations to exercise that are associated with a reduction of fatigue and of physical and psychological stress.

Overloading for Strength

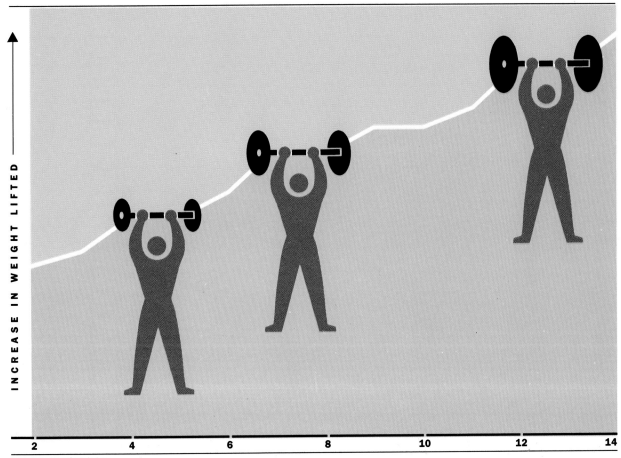

INCREASE IN WEIGHT LIFTED →

Weeks of training

2   4   6   8   10   12   14

neurons, which are the structural and functional units of the system, to the muscle fibers they control *(see illustration page 10)*.

Also, the muscles themselves adapt to the demand being placed on them. With enough training, and with adequate rest between training sessions, the fibers, or individual cells, that make up a muscle actually grow larger by means of a complex process of protein synthesis. This process prompts existing myofibrils — the structures within a muscle that contract — to thicken and new ones to be created.

These changes contribute to the enlargement of the muscle fibers, and thus the increased girth of the muscle itself, in a process known as hypertrophy, the technical term for muscle growth as a result of increased cell size. One study of hypertrophy found that the so-called fast-twitch muscle fibers, which are called into play during activities that require power or sudden bursts of energy, of trained weight lifters were 45 percent larger than those of sedentary people and trained endurance athletes. Accompanying these changes are a number of others, including a thickening of the connective tissues

Overloading muscles with progressively greater amounts of weight, in conjunction with adequate amounts of rest, increases muscle strength. Studies indicate that beginning weight lifters achieve steady gains during the first few weeks of training, as illustrated above. Thereafter, it is common to hit strength plateaus, where gains come more slowly or even level out. Often these plateaus are a result of not properly increasing the overload in accordance with the strength gains, and they can be overcome with a few additional training sessions.

How Strength Starts

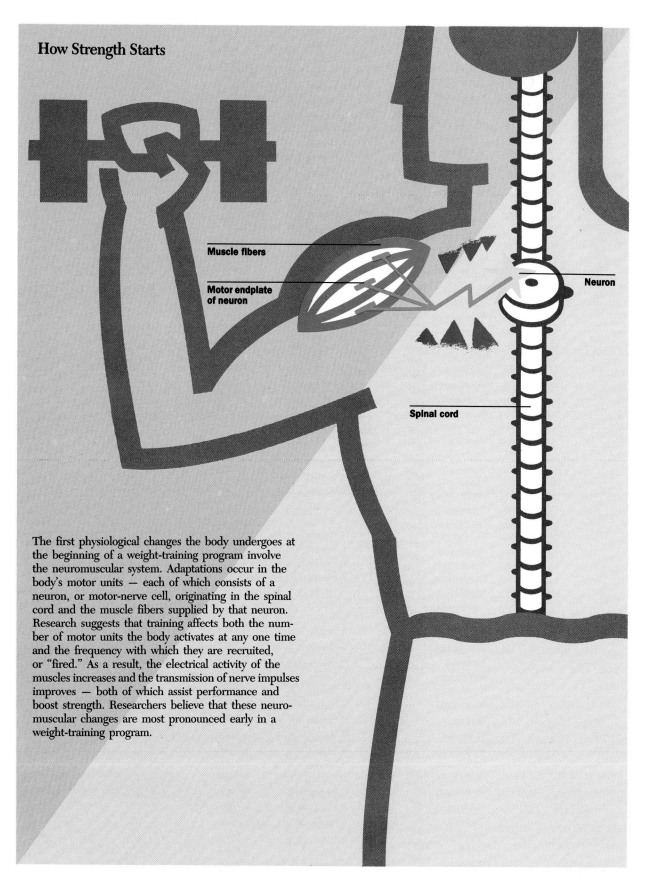

Muscle fibers

Motor endplate of neuron

Neuron

Spinal cord

The first physiological changes the body undergoes at the beginning of a weight-training program involve the neuromuscular system. Adaptations occur in the body's motor units — each of which consists of a neuron, or motor-nerve cell, originating in the spinal cord and the muscle fibers supplied by that neuron. Research suggests that training affects both the number of motor units the body activates at any one time and the frequency with which they are recruited, or "fired." As a result, the electrical activity of the muscles increases and the transmission of nerve impulses improves — both of which assist performance and boost strength. Researchers believe that these neuromuscular changes are most pronounced early in a weight-training program.

that surround muscles and of the tendons that attach muscles to bones. Ligaments, which attach bone to bone, are also strengthened, thus improving joint stability. In addition, weight training produces an increase in glycogen and other energy-releasing compounds within muscle cells. This intracellular activity, along with a decrease in intra-muscular fat, enables the muscles to contract more efficiently for greater strength and endurance.

How does strength differ from muscular endurance?

Strength is generally defined by physiologists as the maximum force a muscle can exert, while endurance is a muscle's ability to keep moving continually without fatigue. Technically, these two elements of fitness are dependent on different muscle-fiber types. Strength is largely a function of a muscle s fast-twitch fibers, so named because they contract rapidly when electrically stimulated. Fast-twitch fibers can rely on the body's anaerobic (without oxygen) energy system when generating powerful contractions for a brief period, which is essential to activities like sprinting and heavy lifting. Endurance is a function of a muscle's slow-twitch fibers, which sustain activities like distance running and cycling, and which are fueled by aerobic (oxygen-supplied) energy.

Both strength and endurance are important components of muscular fitness, and the evidence suggests that training for one will somewhat enhance the development of the other. For example, the person who has built up strength in his lower legs will have more endurance for long-distance running than one whose workout lacks a leg-strengthening component. In a weight-training program, physiologists believe that the key to developing strength is lifting weight that closely approaches your maximum capability — which also tends to build muscle mass. Endurance, on the other hand, is built by performing many repetitions of an exercise — perhaps 20 or more — with less weight. For those starting a weight-training program, it is best to work at building both strength and endurance, and the guidelines on pages 20-21 explain how to do this.

How does weight training develop your physique?

More important to most exercisers than achieving massive bulk is the muscle sculpting that weight training produces. Though any weight-training program should include all the body's major muscles, the use of weights allows you to target those muscles that are weakest and to enhance their size and shape to bring them into pleasing proportion with other body parts. Moreover, if you control your intake of calories, weight training can help trim subcutaneous body fat, which can otherwise obscure a muscle's shape. Pound for pound, muscle burns more calories than fat, but muscle is more compact, occupying 20 percent less space. The end result is a stronger and more efficient, though not necessarily larger, body.

Does weight training offer aerobic fitness benefits?

In many health clubs, machines are arranged in a sequence, or circuit, and some trainers have claimed that by moving quickly through a machine circuit, it is possible to raise your heart rate to the point where you get aerobic benefits for your cardiovascular system. However, most researchers believe that because weight training demands only short bursts of power by specific muscle groups, rather than continuously working large muscles, it contributes little to improving cardiovascular efficiency, which is indicated by a lower resting heart rate, among other signs. A study of Belgian Olympic weight lifters found that while these men possessed a high level of strength, their levels of aerobic fitness were about the same as those of the general population.

An aerobic-training program to benefit the cardiovascular system involves sustained activity by the body's large muscles for at least 20 minutes at a stretch — running, biking or brisk walking, for example. Therefore, a weight-training program should be performed in addition to regular aerobic exercise.

Can weight training make you overly developed or "muscle-bound"?

The image of the rigid, hulking weight lifter is a stereotype based on misconceptions of what muscle growth and strength involve. Competitive body builders typically train intensely for several hours five or six days a week, and it often takes them years to achieve their extreme muscle size and definition. Perhaps more important, physiologists now agree that intense training can do only so much; successful body builders and competitive weight lifters have genetic endowments that aid their prodigious development. Research has also shown that weight training does not impair flexibility, nor does it hamper coordination. In fact, properly performed weight training has been shown to enhance flexibility and coordination in athletes.

If heredity plays a role, how much can the average person achieve with weight training?

A realistic expectation for the average person is an increase in strength of at most five percent a week for the first few weeks — and a smaller percentage increase in the following weeks and months — as well as a modest increase in muscle size, or girth *(see chart opposite)*. If rounded, sloped shoulders tend to run in your family, for example, conditioning your upper body will not completely alter those contours, but adding muscle mass will help compensate.

Can women expect the same results as men?

Women — even female body builders — do not develop the bulging muscles attainable by men for one simple reason: Females produce only a small fraction of the hormone testosterone that males do, and researchers believe that this hormone may promote the building of

Muscle Building in Men and Women

**Muscle size
increase in inches**

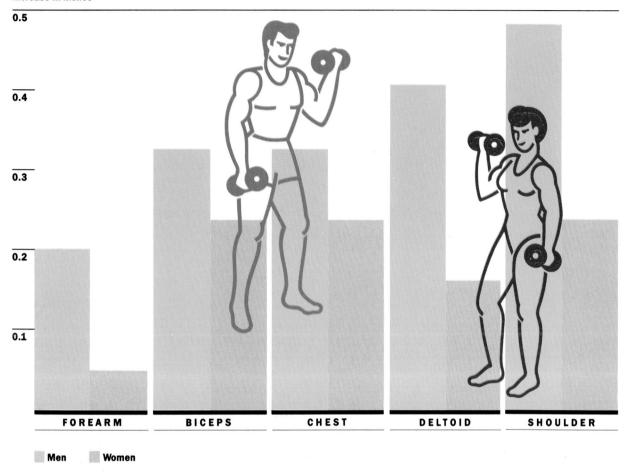

FOREARM	BICEPS	CHEST	DELTOID	SHOULDER

■ Men ■ Women

muscle mass. As a result, women can participate in weight training with no fear that they will "bulk up" like a man, but with every expectation of improved muscle definition and strength.

In fact, while one study found that women are only about two thirds as strong as men in absolute strength, the male advantage virtually disappears when strength is calculated taking body size and composition into account. When strength is instead measured in terms of muscle, rather than overall body weight, women actually come out stronger than men in the legs and hips. Weight-trained women have achieved strength gains equal to and even greater than improvements achieved by men.

Does working with weights slow the inevitable loss of strength that accompanies age?
Both men and women reach their peak of strength in their twenties, on the average, and tend to decline in strength thereafter; however,

Women can gain substantial strength through weight training, but they do not gain muscle bulk to the extent that men do. One study, illustrated above, compared increases in muscle size in both sexes. After an intensive 10-week training regimen, the two groups experienced similar gains in strength, but men gained more muscle mass at five key points. Researchers attribute this difference to the hormone testosterone, which is 10 times more abundant in men than in women.

Lifting and Lowering

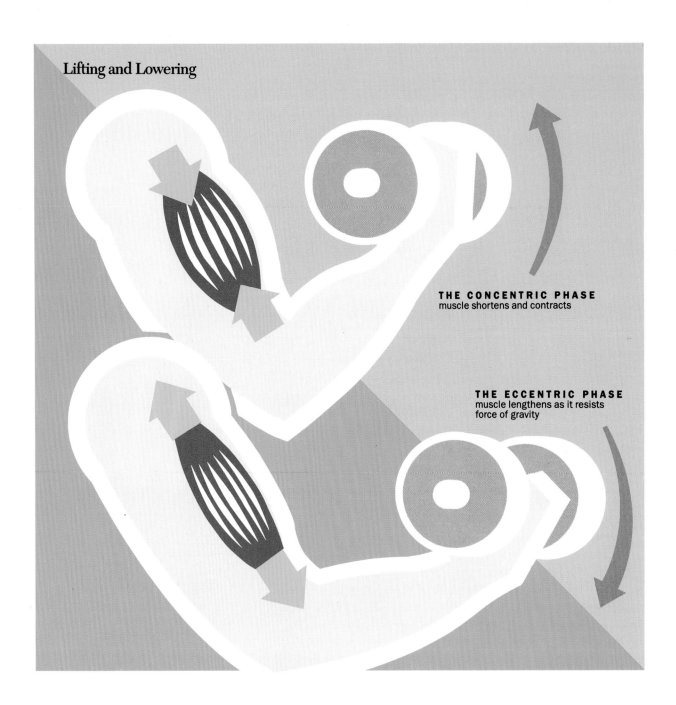

THE CONCENTRIC PHASE
muscle shortens and contracts

THE ECCENTRIC PHASE
muscle lengthens as it resists
force of gravity

You strengthen muscles not only when you lift a weight — which causes a concentric contraction, as illustrated above — but during the lowering phase as well, when the muscles lengthen at a controlled rate as they try to prevent the weight from falling. Exercising to place maximum stress on muscles during this lowering, or eccentric, phase is known as negative loading, which can be used to strengthen muscles further, as shown in the graph opposite.

this fall-off can be modified at any time by effective conditioning. In other words, through training you can outperform the projected level of strength for your age and sex. If you are middle-aged or older, you can achieve the strength level of an untrained younger person.

Can weight training help you lose weight?
Training with free weights or machines will not produce the same kind of weight loss that an aerobic exercise program will provide, because it will not use up calories as quickly. Rather than shedding

pounds, participants in weight-training programs often experience an increase in muscle. The new body shape that emerges is likely to be firmer, more shapely and slimmer-looking, even though body weight may stay unchanged — or even rise slightly, because muscle tissue is heavier than fat tissue. And since muscle burns calories at a higher rate than does body fat, adherence to a weight-training or other exercise program may make it possible to maintain your weight without having to diet. In one study of sedentary middle-aged women who began weight training, the average change in body composition was a shift of nine pounds of fat to nine pounds of muscle. Despite the constancy in the weight of the participants, who were told not to go on a reduced-calorie diet, the women's measurements decreased by an average of 1.25 inches on their hips and 1.0 inches at the waist, and they gained 0.5 inches in their busts on average.

Which type of training will produce the better gains — free weights or machines?

Neither method of training has been proven to be better. The free weight approach is generally favored by body builders and serious weight lifters, and it can produce impressive gains in strength and muscle mass. It can also help build motor coordination, since using free weights requires balance, careful body placement and attention to both the lifting and lowering phases of an exercise. Machines, on the other hand, are safer and easier to use than free weights, and the newer ones have been designed to provide maximum stress throughout a muscle's range of motion, which free weights cannot do. The following chapters cover in detail the benefits and limitations of each type of system.

Can anyone undertake a weight-training program?

Those with a high risk of heart disease or with existing cardiovascular disease are generally advised to stay away from weight training, or to proceed only with their doctor's approval. Intense muscle exertion can cause a temporary rise in blood pressure, which can be dangerous to individuals in high-risk groups. Training with heavy weights can cause you to hold your breath while lifting, which can create pressure in the chest cavity, affecting the veins that return blood to the heart, and raising blood pressure even further. Otherwise, there are no restrictions on weight training for adults, and you can begin a program no matter what your present level of fitness. For guidelines on setting up your own program, turn the page.

Strength and Negative Loading

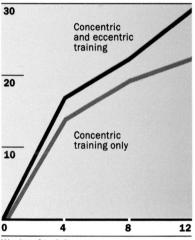

% Strength gain

Concentric and eccentric training

Concentric training only

Weeks of training

Negative loading requires using more weight than you can lift without the help of a partner for the eccentric, or lowering, phase of an exercise. The extra weight is necessary because lowering is aided by gravity and so eases the demand on muscles. The graph above shows the results of a 12-week program in which subjects performed squatting exercises for their leg muscles. Subjects who spent half their training time performing negative-loaded exercises made greater strength gains than those who kept the weight equal during an exercise.

How to Design Your Own Program

All the exercises in the following chapters are aimed at strengthening and shaping muscles. But before you start any workout with weights, you should assess your goals, including what muscle groups you want to concentrate on and where you want to exercise. Begin by answering the questions on these two pages. Then go over the material on the following six pages, which cover the major muscle groups, the basic training terms and guidelines and the warm-ups you should perform.

What are your training goals?

1 **Do you want to be stronger?**

The ability to lift your own weight, for instance when you perform a push-up or chin-up, is a standard gauge of muscular strength. According to the President's Council on Physical Fitness, nine in 10 Americans cannot complete one push-up or chin-up.

Regardless of the level you start from, the workouts in Chapters Two and Three will help you strengthen all your major muscle groups. If you are a beginner, you may notice an improvement within a few weeks. Not only will you soon be able to lift your own weight, but you will find that you can carry ordinary objects — from suitcases to bags of groceries — with greater ease.

2 **Is your lower body firmer and better defined than your upper body?**

If so, then you are among the vast majority of people whose muscular development and tone in their legs is far better than in their arms, shoulders, back and abdomen. Studies have shown that the upper body is the most neglected area; however, for this very reason the muscles in your upper body may respond the most quickly to training efforts.

3 **Are your muscles hidden by body fat?**

Weight lifting is one of the most effective ways to shape and tone muscles. But such a program does not require a considerable expenditure of energy in the form of calories. The best way to sculpt your body so that your muscular development is noticeable is by using weight training in conjunction with regular aerobic exercise to burn calories. Activities like running, cycling and swimming require you to expend energy at a relatively high rate. When aerobic exercise is combined with a well-balanced eating plan, you are likely to lose some of the excess fat you may have acquired through inactivity, overeating or both. The muscles you develop and define by weight training will then become evident.

4 **Do you work out regularly at some other kind of exercise?**

If so, you have already conditioned some of your body's muscle groups. But do not assume that such conditioning will carry over to weight training. Distance runners, for example, build up muscular endurance in their legs, but they may have barely enough strength to lift a weight for a few repetitions. Similarly, although swimming is an excellent upper-body conditioner, its specific movements and the type of resistance it provides do not prepare muscles for exercises with weights. If you are in good shape overall but a newcomer to weight training, be prepared to start at a beginning level and to experience some muscle soreness after the first few workouts.

5   Would you prefer to work out at home?

A set of dumbbells, a barbell with removable weighted plates and an exercise bench are all that you need to start a weight-training program at home. This equipment, available at most sporting goods stores, will allow you as much variety as you need to begin conditioning your entire body. Chapter Two provides specific information on what to buy and how to perform a basic workout.

6   Do you belong to — or do you wish to join — a gym or health club?

For many people, the convenience of working out at home is counterbalanced by some limitations. A good fitness center has more elaborate and often newer, state-of-the-art equipment than anything you can purchase for yourself. Some of the machines, like those used in Chapter Three, are safer and easier to use than free weights. You may also find partners at a club who can enhance your motivation and help ensure your safety when you lift free weights. Usually, at commercial gyms and health clubs, trained staff members who can offer you their expertise are available. Identifying your goals and knowing your own exercise habits will help you weigh the advantages and disadvantages of the home and gym workouts.

7   Should you eat a special diet?

There is no scientific evidence to support the dietary practice of many body builders, who consume extra protein — 40 percent, or even more, of their total calories daily. The only way to strengthen muscles is through a regular program of exercise that overloads, or taxes, the muscles, thereby increasing the size of existing muscle fibers. The recipes in Chapter Five provide dishes that follow nutritionally sound guidelines for protein intake — 15 percent of the total daily calories you consume.

Can steroids help?

One way that body builders and other athletes reputedly increase their muscle mass is by taking anabolic steroids — drugs that function in a manner similar to testosterone, the male hormone chiefly responsible for muscle growth. Some studies have shown strength gains with steroid use in men who exercise; however, there is mounting evidence that steroids produce serious side effects far outweighing any possible gains.

Steroid use has been shown to interfere with testosterone production in men and the menstrual cycle in women, and to damage the liver and reproductive system in both sexes. Perhaps most surprising, it also produces a rapid lowering of HDL cholesterol, the form that appears to help ward off heart disease.

Forearm
pages 50, 51, 114, 115

Biceps
pages 46, 47, 77, 106–109

Pectorals
pages 42, 70–73, 94–97

Abdominals
pages 52, 53, 116, 117, 119

Obliques
pages 53, 65

Hip flexors
pages 77, 78, 87

Abductors
pages 36, 37, 62

Adductors
pages 36, 37, 63

Quadriceps
pages 32–34, 60, 84–89

Shaping Your Body

A sound weight-training program should condition all your major muscles. But you may want to give certain body parts extra attention. Use the illustrations at right to identify the muscle groups; the page references will direct you to exercises that will develop those groups. To promote muscle balance, be sure to include exercises for opposing muscle groups. If you train the quadriceps on the front of your thighs, for instance, you should also train the hamstrings on the back of your thighs. For a more complete workout, use the routines in Chapters Two or Three.

Whatever exercises or training method you choose, be sure to read the following four pages in order to perform the exercises effectively.

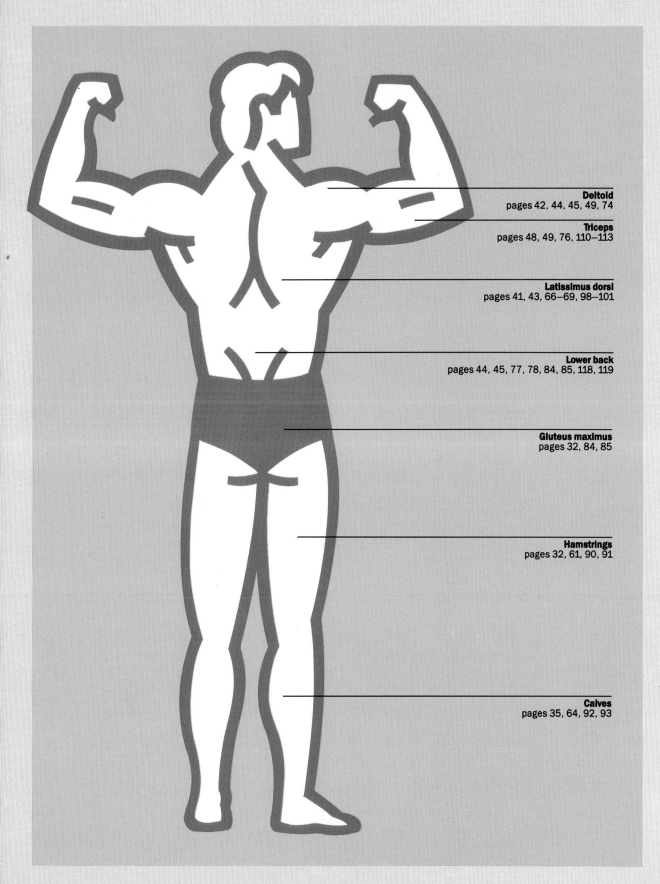

Deltoid
pages 42, 44, 45, 49, 74

Triceps
pages 48, 49, 76, 110–113

Latissimus dorsi
pages 41, 43, 66–69, 98–101

Lower back
pages 44, 45, 77, 78, 84, 85, 118, 119

Gluteus maximus
pages 32, 84, 85

Hamstrings
pages 32, 61, 90, 91

Calves
pages 35, 64, 92, 93

Training Terms

Repetition. Often abbreviated as *rep,* a repetition is one complete sequence of a single exercise. It is the basic unit of all weight-training exercises. To perform a biceps curl for 10 reps means that you lift a dumbbell or barbell from your waist to your shoulders 10 times.

Set. A set is a fixed number of repetitions. To perform a biceps curl for two sets of 10 repetitions, you must curl the weight 10 times, rest for a minute or so, and then perform 10 more curls.

Training to failure. Building muscles according to the overload principle means making them work progressively harder. One way to do this is to train them to failure. Stimulate the muscles maximally to improve strength by stressing them with enough weight during a set so that the last repetition is fairly difficult. If you are doing sets of 10, for instance, you should feel that you could not complete an 11th rep.

Negative reps. Exercises involving eccentric contractions, during which a muscle lengthens while resisting force, are called negative reps. To intensify your workout by performing negative reps, you must lower a weight that is heavier than one you can raise for the equivalent exercise. Although you can do some negative exercises on your own, you will usually need a partner to help you raise the weight again. Do not perform negative work if you are a beginner; only experienced lifters should do negative reps. Once you have progressed to the advanced exercises in Chapter Four, add one or two negative exercises to your regular workout. Do them no more than once a week.

Range of motion. A muscle's range of motion is the entire arc through which it can move. While lifting weights or using exercise machines, try to move the muscle being worked through its entire range of motion in order to ensure more complete strength development.

Planning Your Regimen

Training objectives. Before you embark on a strength-training program, determine your goals. In addition to increasing your muscle tone and definition, do you want to improve your muscular endurance? Or are you interested primarily in increasing your strength? Although most weight-training programs will improve both your strength and endurance, generally speaking, if you want to emphasize endurance, you should lift light weights for a high number of reps. To emphasize strength, you should go for few reps but lift close to your maximum load. To increase your strength and endurance, you should lift an intermediate amount of weight for a moderate number of reps.

How much weight. Once you have determined your goals in a weight-lifting program, you should find out how much weight you can lift in a single repetition. This will take some experimentation. Since you will be lifting a weight at your maximum ability, you should have a partner stand by as a spotter in case you lose control.

To develop both strength and endurance, you should then try to lift about 75 to 85 percent of the maximum weight you can handle. (If you can lift 100 pounds once, for example, you should work out with 75 to 85 pounds.) To develop strength, you should lift weights amounting to about 80 to 90 percent of your maximum; for endurance, you should lift about 55 to 75 percent of your maximum. Over time, you will be able to use your experience and your instincts to judge how much weight you need.

How many reps. To develop strength, you should lift 80 to 90 percent of your maximum weight in a set of three to six repetitions. To train for endurance, lift 55 to 75 percent of your maximum for as many repetitions as you can — as many as 20 or even 40. Those training for both strength and endurance should aim to complete three sets of 10 to 15 repetitions.

Increasing the weight. Weight training involves progressive resistance. Once you can perform more than the specified reps of a particular exercise during two consecutive workout sessions, increase the weight by five percent.

Frequency. Try to exercise three times a week. You should get no less than 48 hours' rest between each workout to allow the muscles to recover. For best results, you should not rest longer than 96 hours between workouts. For example, you can work out on Mondays, Wednesdays and Fridays, resting on Tuesdays, Thursdays and weekends.

If you wish, you may divide your workout schedule into alternate days of lower body and upper body routines. For instance, you can do a lower body workout on Mondays, Wednesdays and Fridays, and an upper body routine on Tuesdays, Thursdays and Fridays.

Guidelines for Working Out

WARM UP.

Perform a five- or 10-minute aerobic warm-up. Most commercial gyms feature stationary bicycles, treadmills, and rowing and cross-country ski machines; these are excellent for warming up. You can also jump rope or jog in place. Warming up will improve blood flow, nerve conduction and flexibility. It will help prevent muscle soreness and reduce the chance of injury as well.

BREATHE NATURALLY.

Holding your breath can lead to a rise in blood pressure, dizziness and fainting, which can be dangerous while lifting heavy weights. Instead, breathe normally through your mouth and nose in rhythm with your exercise. Complete a breath cycle with each rep: Exhale while you lift a weight and inhale while you lower it. During some exercises that require a stable chest — such as a bench press — you may be tempted to take a deep breath and hold it. Instead, continue to exhale as you lift and contract your abdominal muscles to stabilize your chest.

AVOID MUSCULAR TENSION.

Relax those muscles not involved with the lift. Focus on the muscles you are exercising and involve only them. Do not tense your face or clench your fists. Creating tension in body parts other than the one you are exercising will take away energy you need for the exercise and needlessly increase your blood pressure.

WORK LARGE MUSCLES FIRST.

If you have not divided your workout into separate upper and lower body routines, begin with the thighs and lower legs, then move on to the chest and back, shoulders, upper arms and forearms, and conclude with the abdominals and lower back. If you tire your small muscles early in the workout by exercising them first, they will not be able to assist as stabilizing muscles when you work your larger muscles. Follow the routine in Chapter Two for a basic free-weight workout that covers all of the major muscle groups. You can use this routine either in a home gym or a commercial facility. If you are working out on machines, follow the routine in Chapter Three.

MAINTAIN MUSCLE BALANCE.

When exercising one muscle group, be sure to exercise the opposing muscle group. This will ensure good muscle balance and may protect against injury. For instance, if you work the biceps, on the top portion of your upper arm, include an exercise for the triceps, on the underside of your upper arm. Similarly, you should work toward bilateral strength — that is, equal conditioning for both sides of your body. When exercising one limb, be sure to repeat the exercise for the other.

INCREASE THE EFFORT.

Once you are familiar with the basic routine in Chapter Two, you can concentrate on certain parts of your body for more intense free-weight exercises. To do that, you can utilize some of the exercises in Chapter Four, which you can add to the basic workout. Many of the exercises in Chapter Four require a partner and the specialized equipment available in commercial gyms.

KEEP A JOURNAL.

Keep track of your progress. For each workout, record in a journal the weights you use, the exercises you employ and the number of sets and reps. This will help you determine how quickly you are progressing and what muscle groups may need more work. Once you have achieved your goals, increasing your work load will not be necessary, but you will have to continue exercising two to three times per week to maintain your fitness.

Warm-Ups and Stretching

Prior to performing any of the conditioning routines presented in this book, you should spend at least five minutes warming up. Simply run in place or do any aerobic exercise that gradually increases your heart rate and metabolism. Many gyms offer stationary bicycles, treadmills, rowing and cross-country skiing machines that provide excellent warm-ups. Studies show that aerobic exercise leads to a rapid temperature rise in the working muscles, which allows them to work faster and more smoothly, improves nerve conduction and increases the supply of oxygen. Warming up before you begin a strength-building regimen will also reduce your risk of injury.

Once you have warmed up, you will feel more "loose" and flexible. This is the best time to begin the strength-building exercises outlined in the following chapters.

After you have completed your workout, you can cool down with a general stretching routine to maintain or improve your overall flexibility. The eight stretches shown at right will increase the range of motion for most of your body's major joints. When performing stretches, do not bounce or jerk your body. Do each stretch slowly and hold it for 15 to 20 seconds. Stretch to the point of discomfort, but not to the point of pain. Remember to stretch both sides of your body; after you stretch the oblique muscles in your right side, for example, as shown at the top of this page, stretch your left side in the same manner.

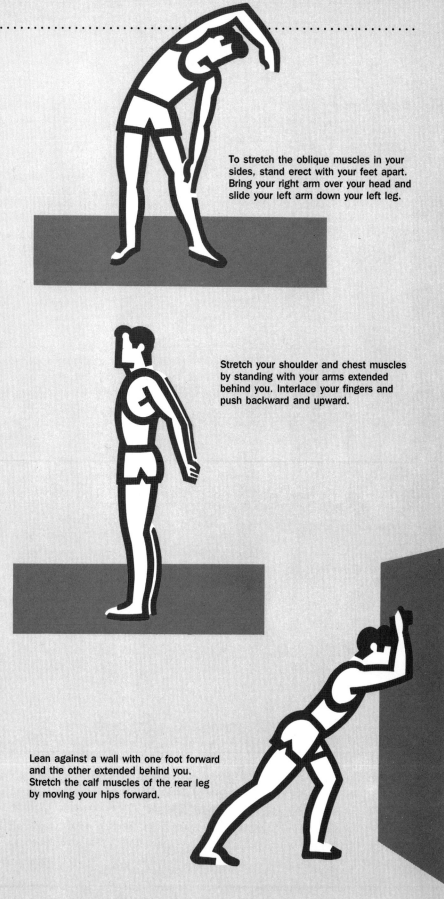

To stretch the oblique muscles in your sides, stand erect with your feet apart. Bring your right arm over your head and slide your left arm down your left leg.

Stretch your shoulder and chest muscles by standing with your arms extended behind you. Interlace your fingers and push backward and upward.

Lean against a wall with one foot forward and the other extended behind you. Stretch the calf muscles of the rear leg by moving your hips forward.

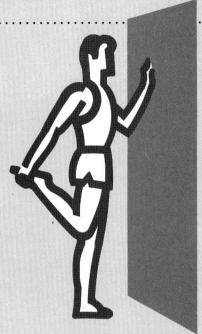

To stretch the quadriceps in the front of your thigh, brace yourself against a wall with one hand and grasp one foot with the other hand. Pull your heel toward your buttocks.

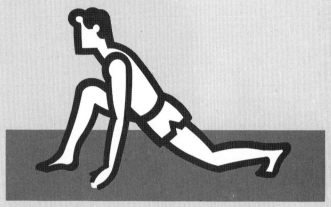

Place your hands on the floor for balance and extend your left foot behind you. Lower your chest toward your right knee and keep your back straight to stretch the hip flexors.

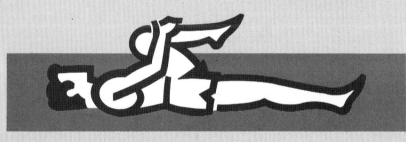

To stretch your hamstrings and lower back, lie on your back with your legs extended. Bring up one knee, grasp it with both hands and draw it toward your chest.

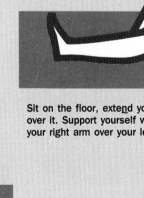

Sit on the floor, extend your right leg and cross your left over it. Support yourself with your left arm; and place your right arm over your left knee. Draw the knee back.

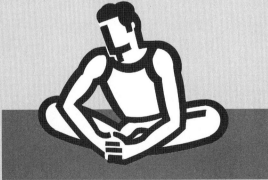

To stretch your lower back and the adductor muscles in your inner thighs, sit on the floor with the soles of your feet together. Grasp your toes and lean forward from the waist.

23

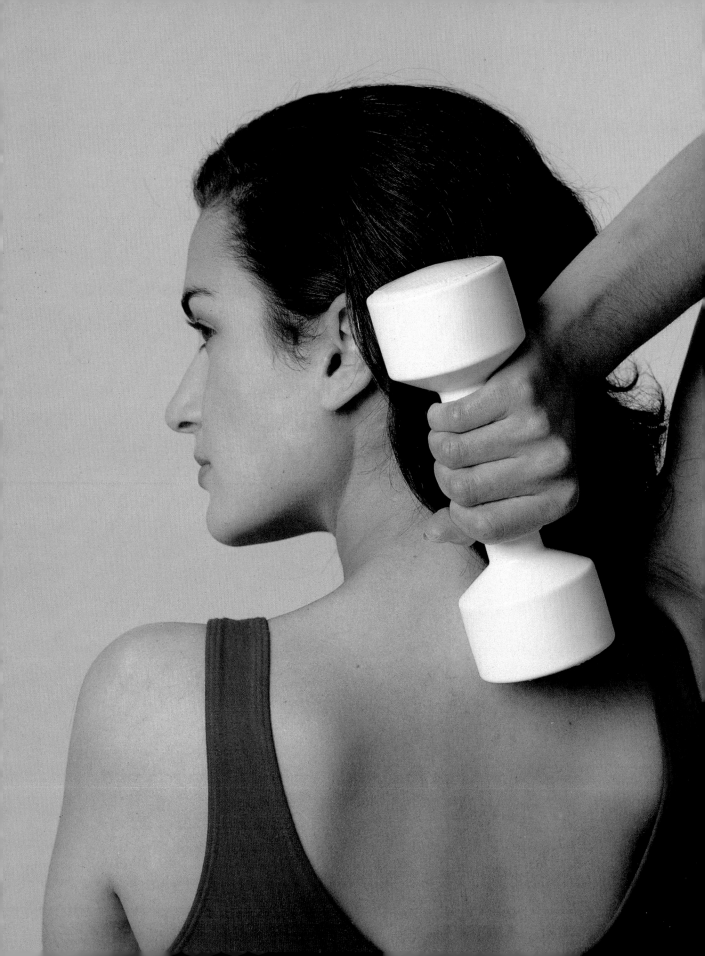

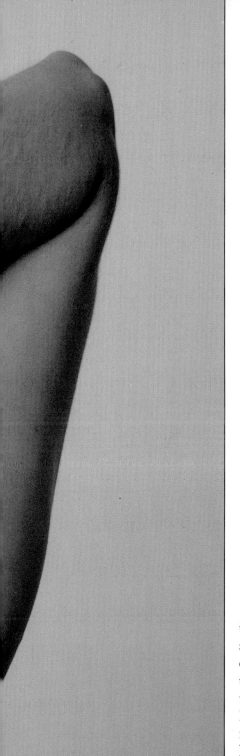

CHAPTER TWO

The Home Gym

The right set-up and a complete workout

The most accessible and effective means to start building up your body through progressive resistance training is by using a basic set of free weights. This consists of dumbbells, a barbell and weighted plates that fit interchangeably on the bar. As you grow stronger, you can add weight to the barbell and use heavier dumbbells to keep your muscles working to the utmost. Furthermore, you can change weights to accommodate different muscle groups: For example, a squatting exercise that will tax the large muscles in your thighs or buttocks requires heavier weights than does an arm curl for your biceps, which are comparatively weaker.

Since the costs of purchasing barbells and dumbbells are relatively low, many people find they can afford to buy the equipment for use at home. The convenience of working out in a home gym is undisputed. Instead of putting aside a whole morning or evening to exercise at a health club or commercial gym, you can save time by working out in the morning before work, right after work or during any leisure time that you may have. In addition to its convenience and the money you may save in health club membership fees, a home gym also allows you to train in private or with friends or family members. You can also listen to music of your choice. All of these advantages can help encourage you to work out regularly.

The start-up costs for a home gym begin at a modest $200 and can go as high as your budget allows. But once you have made that initial investment, there need not be any further costs: You will have all the basic equipment you need for a thorough workout *(pages 28-29)*.

Along with the equipment, you need a place to exercise. You do not need a lot of space — three body builders who won the Mr. America title worked out in a one-car garage — but you should have enough room to move freely, so that you are not distracted by the worry of banging into something with a barbell. If possible, set aside a space that you use only for working out: Packing your equipment away after every workout makes it more likely you will find reasons not to unpack it another time. Also, try to locate your gym in a basement, or on the ground floor of your home, which will provide a solid surface should weights drop on the floor.

Whatever space you use, your home gym should be well ventilated and have a suitable floor surface. Avoid concrete or tile flooring, since these surfaces may be too slippery and unstable. On the other hand, rubberized surfaces provide too much resistance and can feel sticky when you work out on them. Hardwood flooring is a good surface, but carpeted floors with padding are the best of all. Carpets are more comfortable than hard floors, absorb sound better and help compensate for an uneven floor that might make your exercise bench tilt or your dumbbell roll. If you work out on a carpeted floor, clean it periodically to prevent the buildup of bacteria.

Be sure the clothing you wear absorbs perspiration and also allows you full range of movement without binding. Wear enough clothing to keep yourself warm; cold muscles are more likely to be injured than warm muscles. Also, be sure to wear shoes. Not only can you sustain a serious injury should a weight fall on a bare foot, but unsupported arches are subject to undue stress when you work out with weights. Wear comfortable footwear that gives you adequate arch as well as lateral support, such as shoes designed for aerobic dance, tennis or basketball. Shoe designers now offer multi-purpose footwear that is excellent for indoor training.

Although exercising in a home gym gives you greater freedom, it also gives you greater responsibility to take charge of your own workouts. One tool to keep you motivated is a training diary for monitoring of your progress. In a calendar or appointment book, note the exercises you perform, the number of sets and repetitions, and the amount of weight you use. This record will provide solid evidence of gains in strength. Another motivating tool is a mirror, which helps you observe proper technique and also allows you to see that your musculature is developing. Finally, if you can arrange it, work out

Home Gym Safety

◆ With a minimum of expense, you can furnish your home gym with enough equipment to give yourself a complete workout. For safety's sake, though, you should not skimp when buying weight-training equipment or any other exercise device. Before purchasing any equipment, try it out in the store and check to see that it appears sturdy.

◆ When working out in your home gym, you should follow certain precautions to ensure that your equipment is safe . While using a barbell, be sure that you have iron collars or clips on the end of the barbell to hold the weights in place and prevent them from slipping out. If a weight slips off the end of a barbell, it can throw you off balance and possibly cause a back injury or other serious harm to your muscles and joints. Although weight clips perform the same function as collars, iron collars are stronger than clips.

◆ When you work out, be sure that friends and other family members who are not exercising give you plenty of room and stay clear of the weights. Take particular care that pets and children are safely out of the way.

◆ Keep your mind on what you are doing. Concentrate while you are performing an exercise, and pay especially close attention when you load and unload weights.

with a training partner. A partner can help you with the more difficult exercises as well as motivate you to work hard and not miss training sessions.

Since you will not be under the supervision of athletic trainers or other professionals if you work out in a home gym, it is a good idea to have a fitness test administered by a qualified exercise physiologist before engaging in your program. If you have a family history of heart trouble or high blood pressure, or if you are 35 years of age or older and have not exercised regularly in the past two years, you should also have a medical check-up.

The basic workout that follows, which can be completed in less than an hour, includes stretching and mobility routines as well as weight-loaded exercises. In some instances, alternative exercises are presented to add variety to the workout. Performing these exercises will make you stronger and firmer, and, if you work diligently at increasing the resistance, they can increase your muscle tone, especially if you are a beginner.

Remember that the point of body sculpting is to use a sufficient amount of weight to stress muscles for growth and symmetry — the absolute amount of weight you can lift is unimportant. Follow the guidelines on pages 20-21. As you experiment with how much weight you can lift, use this initial training time to concentrate on the technique of lifting. Proper form is crucial for getting the maximum benefit from the overload you are placing on your muscles.

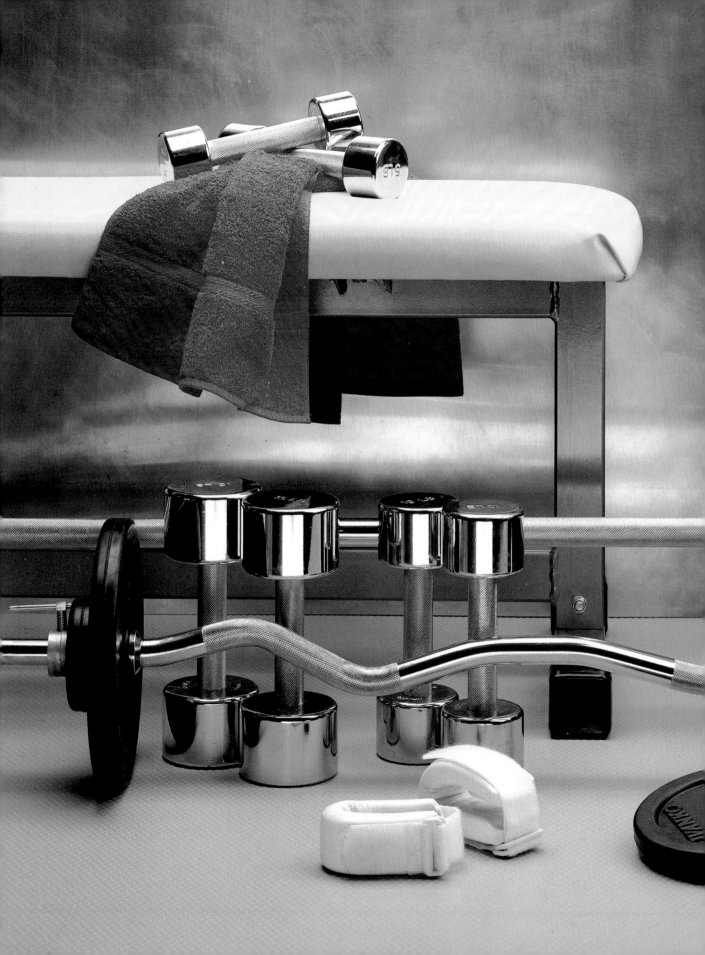

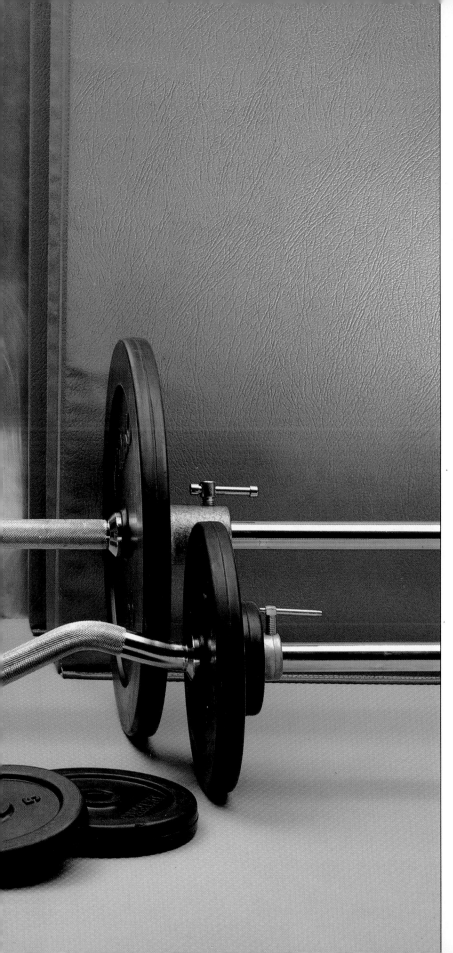

Equipment

The tools you need to outfit a home gym geared toward strength training are shown at left. The two most basic pieces of equipment to buy are a barbell with plates and a set of dumbbells. You should also purchase ankle weights for lower body workouts, an exercise bench to perform certain exercises and an exercise mat, so that you can work out comfortably on the floor.

A barbell is usually a four- to six-foot steel bar that is about an inch in diameter; it can be either solid or hollow. You can slide iron plates over the ends of the bar and use collars or clips to prevent them from sliding off. The plates, sometimes covered with rubber, come in varying weights from 1.25 to 100 pounds. For biceps curls, some people prefer a curling bar, shown in the foreground, to the standard barbell because its shape relieves stress on the forearms.

Dumbbells are simply short barbells, usually 10 to 16 inches long, that you can hold with one hand. You can use dumbbells one at a time or one in each hand simultaneously. There are two kinds of dumbbells. Plate-loaded dumbbells have removable weights; solid dumbbells have weights attached to the ends of the bar. Solid dumbbells can be often purchased in sets of weights ranging from 2.5 to 20 pounds and more.

Lower Body/1

Because your lower body is the site of your largest muscles and some of your most powerful ones, you should start a training session by concentrating on it. Begin with the large muscles in your buttocks and your thighs; working these larger muscle groups before the smaller groups — like those in your calf — helps prevent the smaller muscles from getting fatigued at the start of your workout.

Take at least five minutes to warm up, following the guidelines on page 22. Then start your workout with the exercises on these two pages, which are designed to increase the mobility in your hips and legs. For the free-weight training exercises that begin on page 32, use enough weight so that the first few repetitions are comfortable to perform, but the last few are fairly difficult. For general conditioning, many people find that three sets of 10 to 15 repetitions are most effective. (If you are a beginner, start by doing one set of each exercise.) When an exercise is shown for only one leg or one side of the body, be sure to perform it for both sides of your body.

Lie face up and place a folded towel under your neck to relieve tension in your shoulders. Draw your knees up and grasp them with your hands *(top)*. Slowly pull your knees toward your chest, then pull them to the sides *(center)*. Rotate your knees for 30-45 seconds to improve mobility in your hips *(right)*.

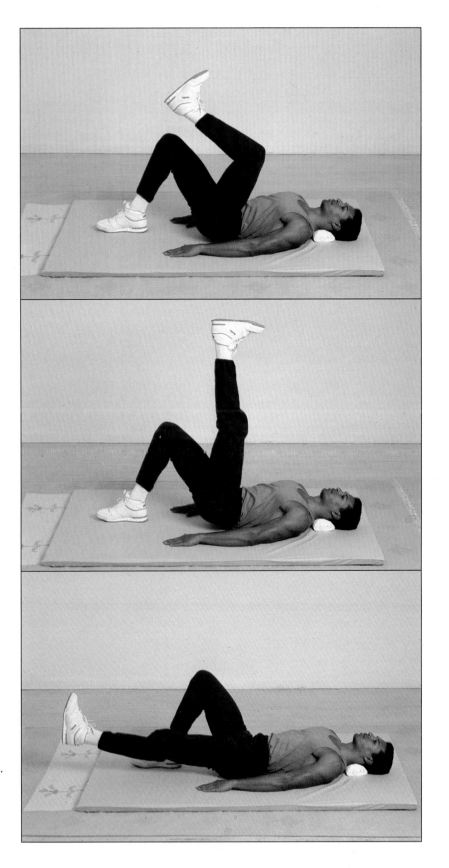

Lie on your back with your right foot flat on the floor and a towel under your neck. Draw your left knee toward your chest *(top)*. Slowly straighten the knee and push your heel toward the ceiling *(center)*. Be sure to keep your hip on the floor. Lower your left leg to the floor slowly *(right)*.

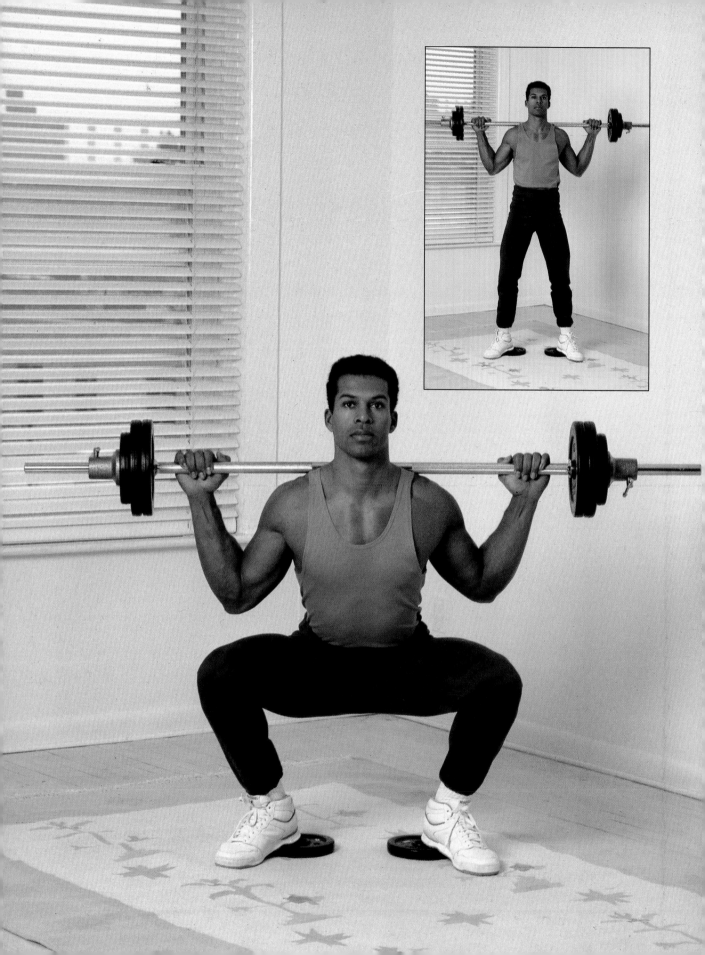

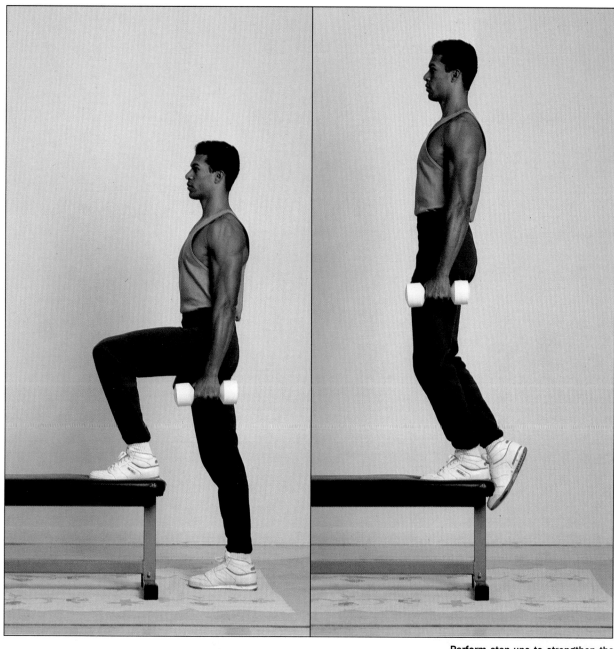

Perform step-ups to strengthen the quadriceps. Place an exercise bench in front of you and hold a 10- to 20-pound dumbbell in your left hand. Looking straight ahead, place your left foot on the bench *(above left)* and step up *(above)*. Do not lock your left knee or place your right foot on the bench. Step down with the right leg, then the left.

Lower Body/2

The squat is the best exercise to develop your thighs and buttocks. Stand with your feet apart and your heels slightly elevated. Place a barbell on your upper back *(inset opposite)*. Keeping your head up, inhale as you lower yourself to a squatting position *(opposite)*. Exhale as you return to the starting position.

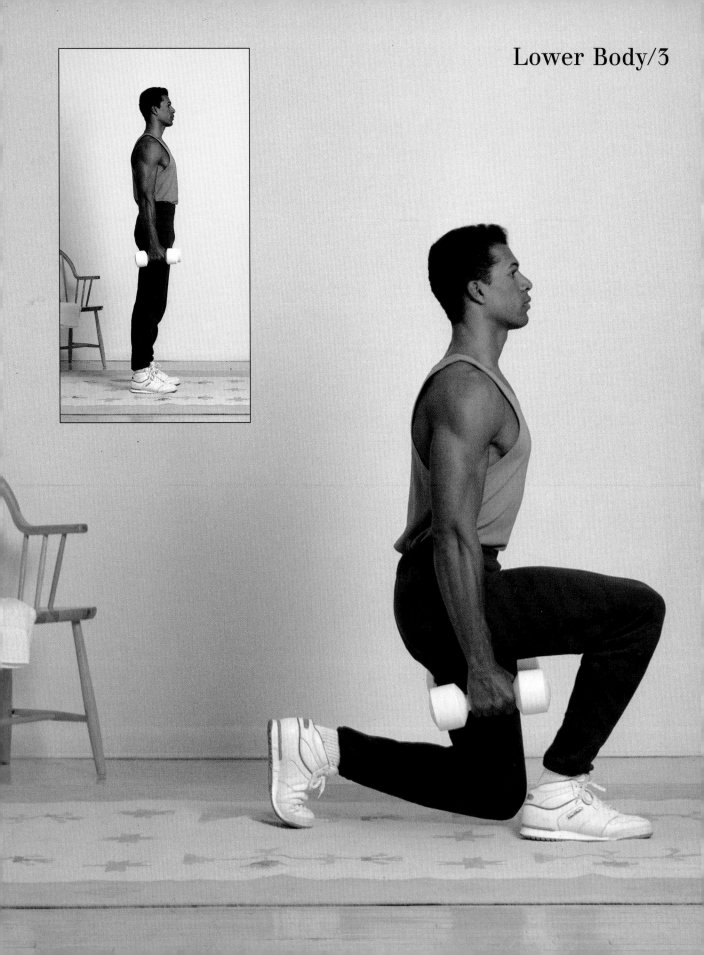

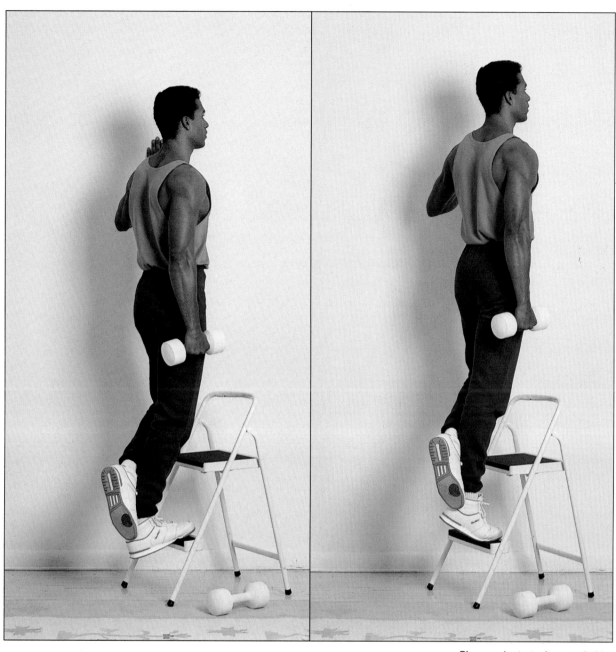

While holding dumbbells, stand erect with your toes pointed forward and your knees straight but not locked *(inset opposite)*. Keeping your head up, step forward with your right foot and drop your left knee to within an inch of the floor *(opposite)*. Be sure that your left knee is just behind your right heel. Then push off the floor with your right foot and return to the starting position. Repeat by stepping forward with your left foot.

Place a short stool or stepladder adjacent to a wall and hold a dumbbell in your right hand. Stand on the first step, your left side facing the wall. Bracing yourself with your left hand on the wall, stand on your right foot and allow your heel to drop as far as it can over the edge of the step. You will feel a stretch in the calf muscle *(above left)*. Lean forward slightly and rise up on the toes of your right foot. Be sure to keep your right leg straight *(above)*.

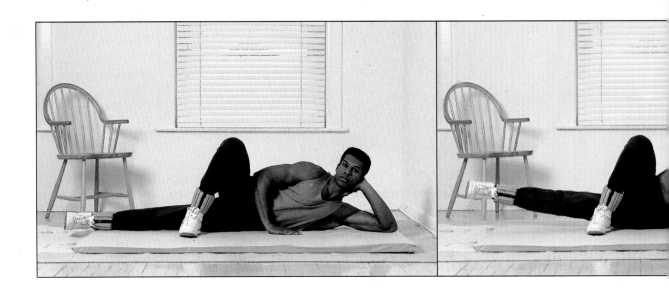

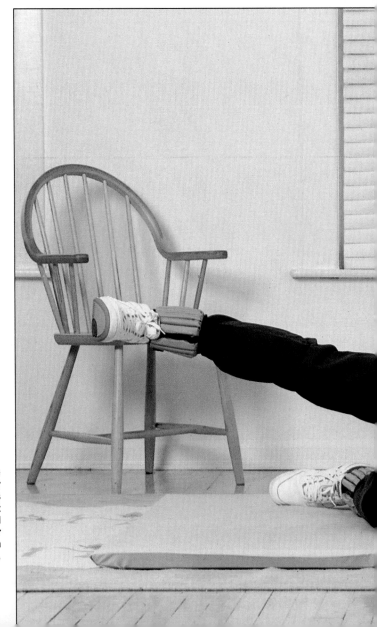

Strengthen the abductors on the outside
of your thighs with an exercise similar
to the one above. Attach ankle weights
and lie on your left side. Bend your left
knee at about a 45-degree angle and
extend your right leg *(inset)*. Raise your
right leg toward the ceiling *(right)*, then
return to the starting position.

Lower Body/4

To strengthen the adductor muscles on your inner thighs, strap on ankle weights and lie on your left side on the floor. Cross your right leg over your left and place your right foot flat on the floor *(far left)*. Keeping your left leg extended, raise it off the floor *(near left)*.

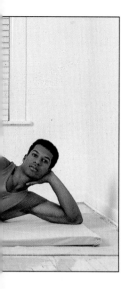

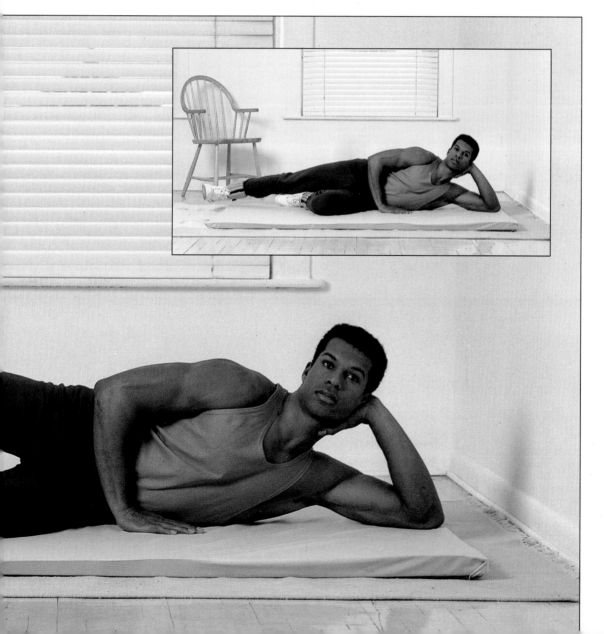

Upper Body/1

Once you have completed the lower body exercises, you can begin working the upper body, which should generally improve your physique as well as restore or maintain good posture. Concentrate on the larger muscles of the chest, back and shoulders before you proceed to the smaller triceps and biceps in the upper arms. Exercise your forearms last, since they contain the smallest muscle groups.

Begin the upper body workout with the mobility and stretching exercises on these two pages and the following two before moving into the strengthening segment. For the weight-training exercises, work up to three sets for each exercise *(see pages 20-21)*. You should be in control of the weights at all times, moving them smoothly and deliberately, never throwing or jerking them. The lowering phase should take as much time as the lifting phase of each exercise.

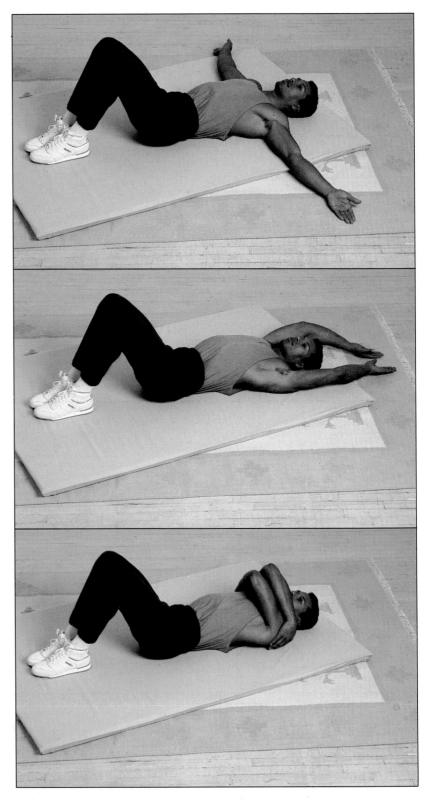

To improve shoulder mobility, lie down with your arms outstretched and your knees bent *(top)*. Slowly move your arms along the floor in an arc until they are above your head *(center)*, cross your arms and lower them over your chest *(right)*, then return to the starting position. This sequence should be one continuous movement. Perform it twice.

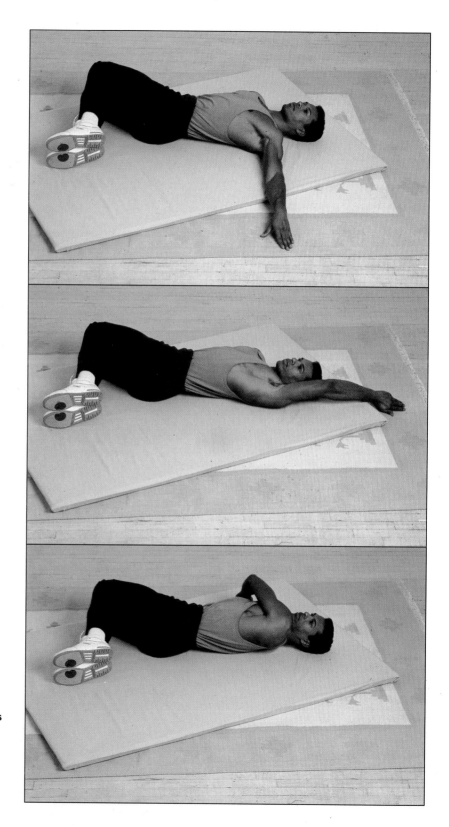

Lie on your back and, keeping both shoulders on the floor, swing your knees to the right until your right knee rests on the floor. Extend your left arm *(top)*. Keeping your hand in contact with the floor, arc your arm above your head *(center)*. Continue arcing *(right)* until you touch your legs. Then perform the exercise in a counterclockwise direction.

Upper Body/2

Perform upper body stretches after your
warm-up or between sets of exercise. To
stretch your chest muscles, stand at
arm's length from a window sill or
doorframe and grasp the corner with
one hand. Turn your body away slightly
but keep your hand in place *(right)*.
Hold for 10 to 20 seconds.

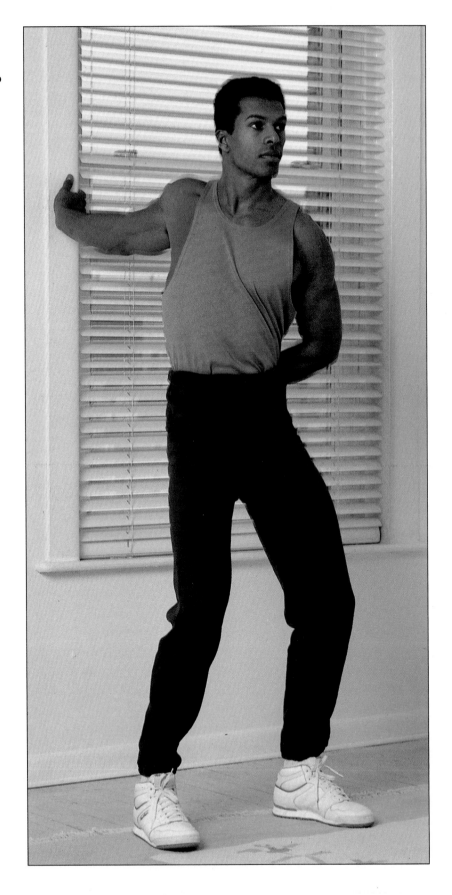

To strengthen your back, lie face up on an exercise bench holding a barbell with your hands shoulder-width apart. Move the weight over and below your head until you feel a stretch in your chest *(right)*. Then contract your upper back and lift the bar until it is just above your chest *(below right)*. Return slowly to the starting position.

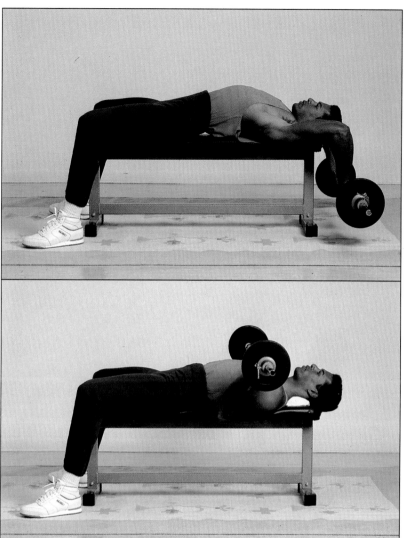

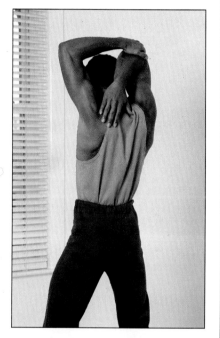

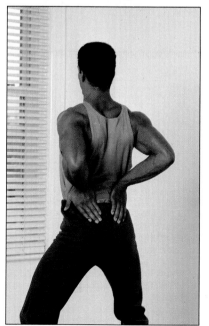

To stretch your triceps muscles, stand or sit erect and raise your right elbow above your head. Grasp it with your left hand and gently but firmly pull it to the left *(above left)*. Hold for 10-20 seconds.

To stretch your shoulder and chest muscles, stand or sit erect and place your hands on the small of your back *(left)*. Squeeze your elbows together and hold for 10-20 seconds.

41

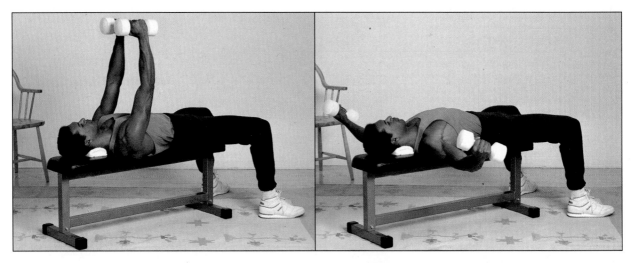

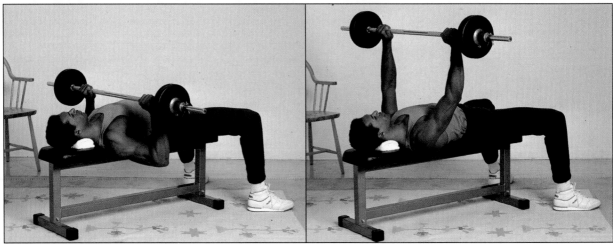

Upper Body/3

Perform bent-arm flys *(top left)* to work your chest and the front of your shoulders. Holding a pair of dumbbells, raise your arms so that the dumbbells are over your chest. Be sure not to lock your elbows. Lower the weights to your sides while inhaling, until you feel a stretch in your chest *(top right).* Contract your chest and bring the dumbbells together while exhaling.

A bench press is similar to a bent-arm fly but also works the triceps. Hold a barbell just above your chest with your hands slightly wider apart than shoulder width *(above left).* Push the weights straight up, but do not lock your elbows *(above right).* Return to the starting position. (For safety, never lift weights near your limit without a partner.)

Perform bent-over rows to strengthen your back and your biceps. Bend over so that your right hand and knee rest on an exercise bench. Keep your left knee bent slightly and dangle a dumbbell in your left hand *(opposite above).* Pull the dumbbell straight up to your chest *(opposite),* keep your elbow close to your body and do not flex your wrist. Return to the starting position.

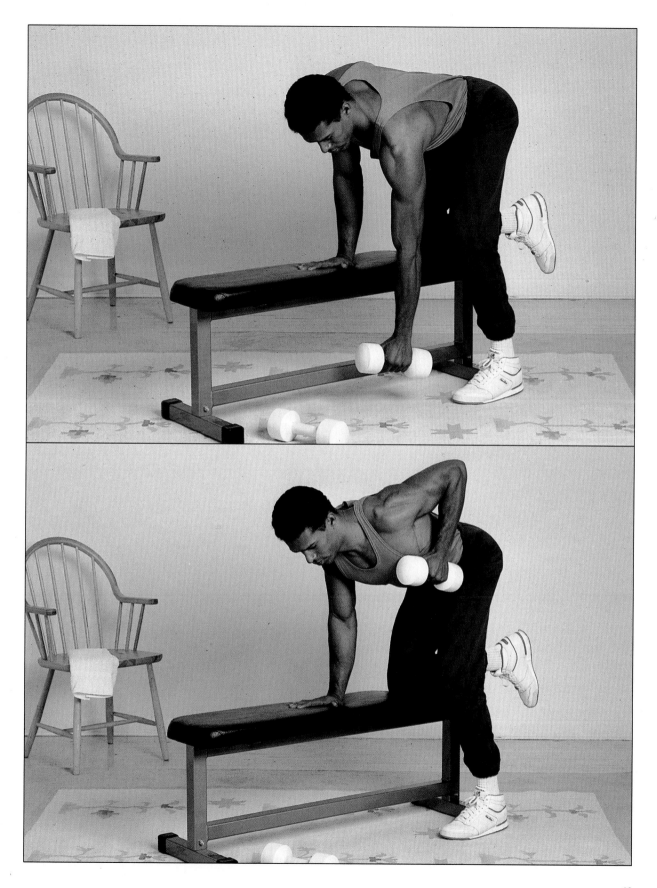

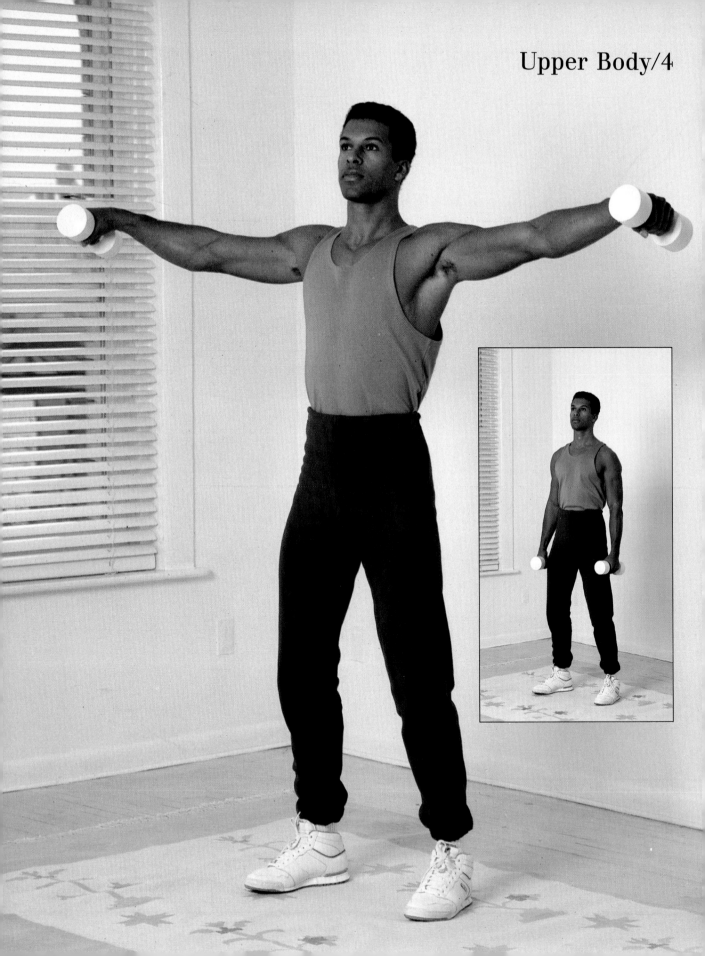

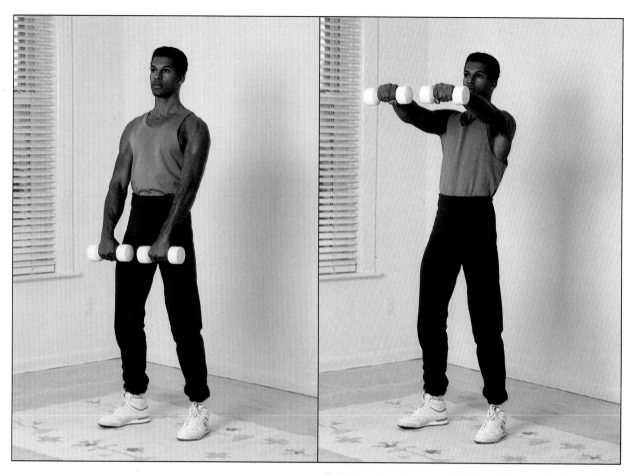

To further strengthen your deltoids, perform anterior arm raises. Standing with your knees slightly bent, hold a pair of dumbbells in front of your thighs with your palms facing inward *(above left)*. Raise the dumbbells until they are at eye level *(above right)*. Return to the starting position.

Perform lateral arm raises to strengthen the deltoid muscles. Stand erect with your knees slightly bent while holding dumbbells at your sides with your palms turned in. Allow the dumbbells to touch your thighs lightly *(inset opposite)*. Tighten your abdominals, keep your knees bent and your back straight, and raise the dumbbells sideways until they are parallel to the floor *(opposite)*. Return to the starting position.

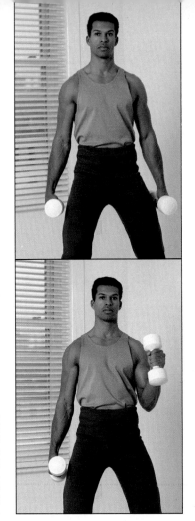

Perform arm curls to shape your biceps. Stand erect with your feet apart and knees slightly bent. Hold dumbbells with your palms facing your outer thighs *(above right)*. Bend your right elbow and raise the dumbbell to chest level *(right)*. Return to the starting position. For this exercise, alternately raise and lower each dumbbell during the set.

Concentration curls are another way to target your biceps. Sit on an exercise bench and stabilize your upper body by resting your left hand on your left thigh. Hold a dumbbell in your extended right arm, resting your right elbow against the inside of your right thigh *(near right)*. Curl the dumbbell to about chest level *(far right)* and then return to the starting position.

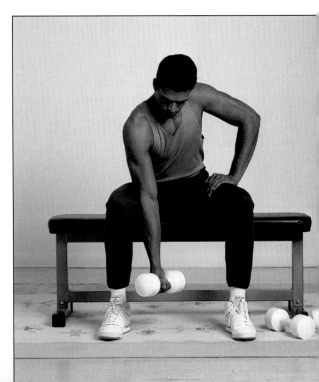

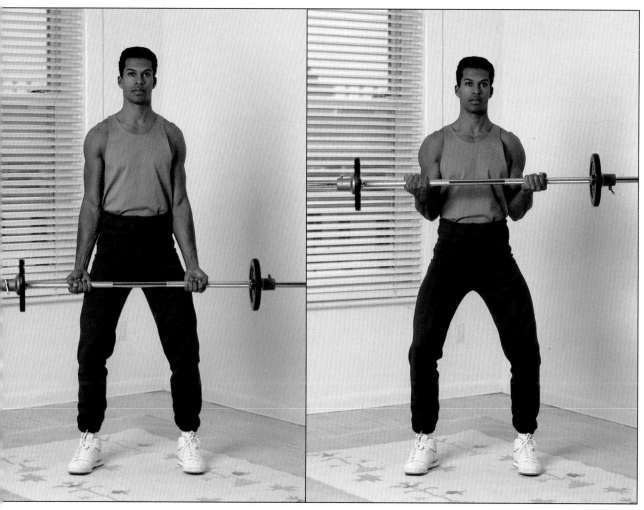

As an alternate to the dumbbell curls, perform arm curls with a weighted barbell or curl bar. Stand erect with your feet apart and your knees slightly bent. Hold the bar with your palms facing forward and about shoulder-width apart *(left)*. Keeping your back straight and head erect, curl the bar to chest level *(right)*. Return to the starting position.

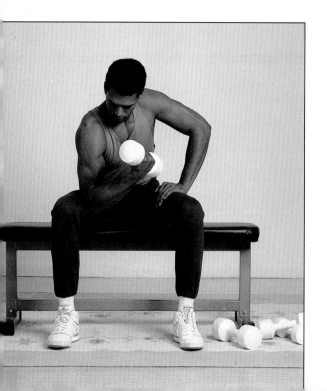

47

Upper Body/6

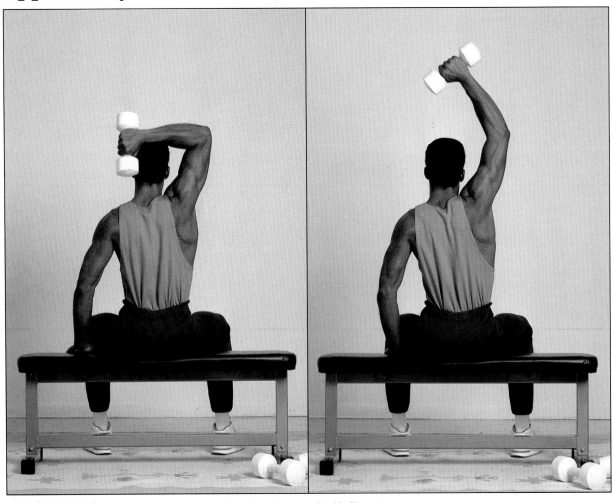

To perform triceps extensions, sit on an exercise bench and grasp a dumbbell in your right hand. Raise the dumbbell over and behind your head. Keep your forearm parallel to the floor *(left).* Straighten your elbow until your arm is extended and the dumbbell is over your head *(right).* Do not lock your elbow or arch your back. Return to the starting position.

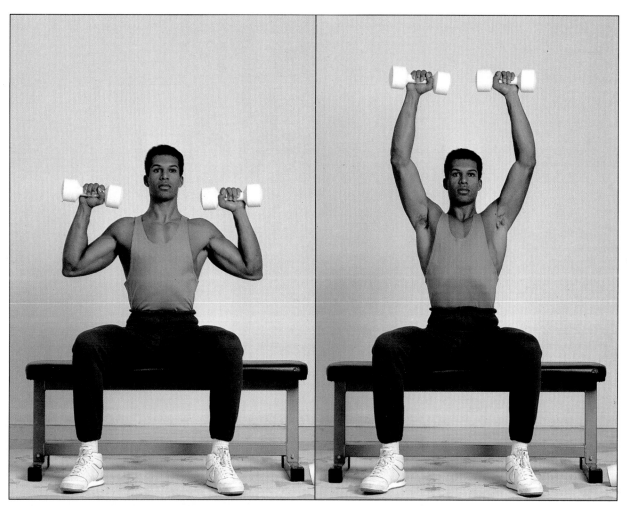

Perform flys for a combination biceps and triceps exercise. Sit on an exercise bench with your back straight and your feet on the floor. Hold two dumbbells at shoulder height with your palms facing forward *(left)*. Imagine that the dumbbells are connected by a bar. Raise them above your head without locking your elbows *(right)*. Return to the starting position.

Upper Body/7

Perform palms-down wrist curls to strengthen the muscles on the inside of your forearms. Kneel over an exercise bench holding a dumbbell in your right hand with your palm down. Rest your left forearm on the bench *(right)*. Raise the dumbbell as high as you can *(bottom right)*. Return to the starting position.

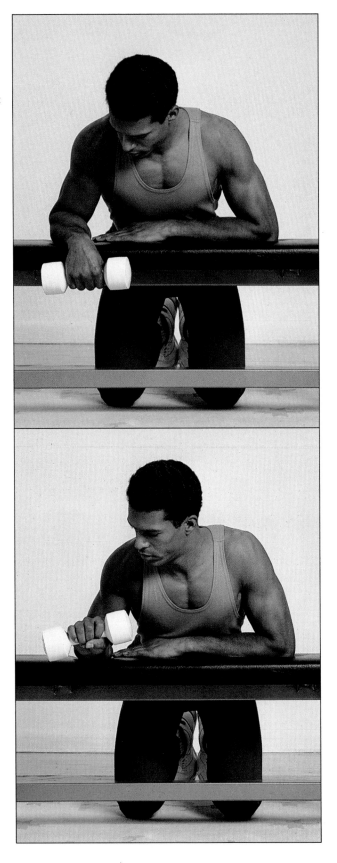

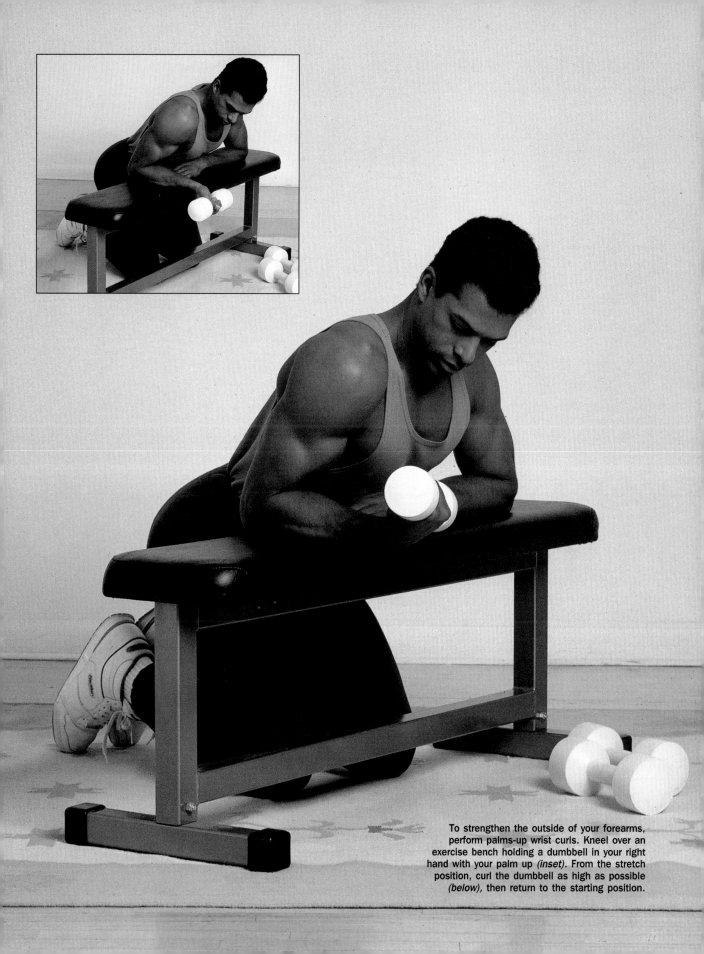

To strengthen the outside of your forearms,
perform palms-up wrist curls. Kneel over an
exercise bench holding a dumbbell in your right
hand with your palm up *(inset)*. From the stretch
position, curl the dumbbell as high as possible
(below), then return to the starting position.

Abdominals and Lower Back/1

Strong, flexible back and abdominal muscles are important for maintaining good posture and avoiding hyperlordosis, or excessive curvature of the spine. If you are like most people, your abdominal muscles are weak in comparison to your opposing back muscles, and you will probably benefit from abdominal muscle strengthening. Because these exercises involve lifting only your own body weight, which remains relatively constant, many body builders perform these exercises with many repetitions per set, often 20-40 or more.

In addition to the benefits to your posture, conditioning these muscles will improve the appearance of your midsection.

Your abdominals and the muscles of your lower back complement each other. When you perform exercises for one group, you should also work to strengthen the other. The exercises on these two pages are intended to strengthen the abdominals, while those on the following two pages will improve the strength of your lower back. If you have a history of back trouble or back pain, do not perform these exercises.

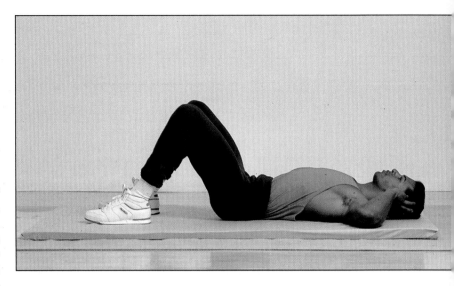

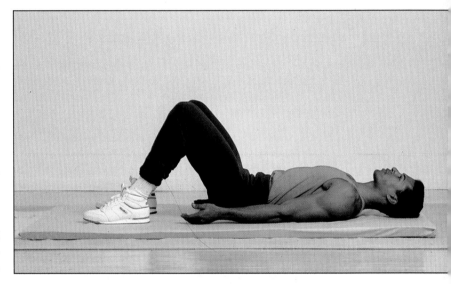

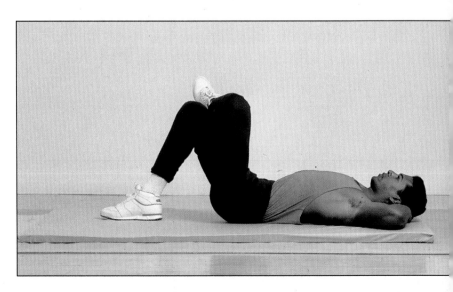

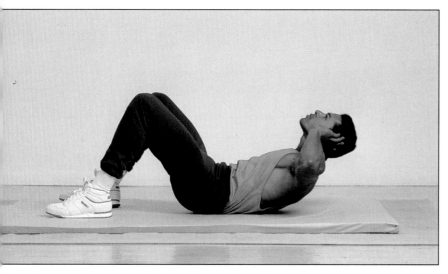

Strengthen your abdominals by performing half sit-ups. Lie on your back with your knees bent, your feet flat on the floor and your fingers intertwined behind your head *(far left)*. Keeping your elbows back, lift your shoulders and upper back off the floor *(left)*. Return to the starting position.

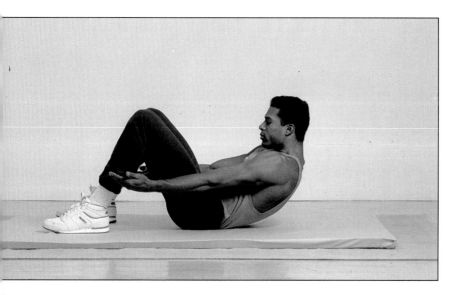

For a more strenuous abdominal exercise, perform curl-ups. Lie on your back, this time with your arms extended down your sides and your palms up *(far left)*. Contract your abdominals and slowly roll your head and upper body up into a half sit-up *(left)*. Return to the starting position.

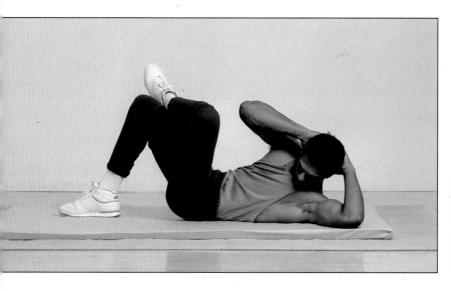

To emphasize the obliques — the side muscles — perform cross-over sit-ups. Lying on your back, lace your fingers behind your head and cross your left foot over your right knee *(far left)*. Keeping your left elbow on the floor, raise your right shoulder and upper back *(left)*. Return to the starting position.

Abdominals and Lower Back/2

To strengthen your lower back muscles, lie face down on the floor with your hands at your sides *(below)*. Raise your chest and shoulders off the floor but keep your pelvis in place *(bottom)*. Hold this position for a few moments, then return slowly to the starting position. Perform the exercise five to 10 times.

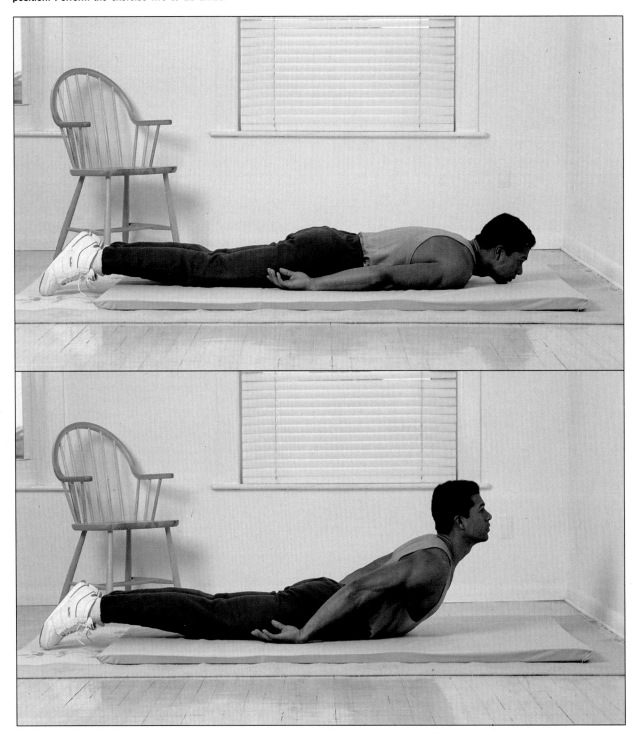

To target your lateral back muscles, lie face down on the floor with your right arm at your side, your left hand resting on the small of your back and your head turned to the left *(below)*. Lift your chest off the floor *(bottom)*. Then return slowly to the starting position. Repeat five to 10 times for each side.

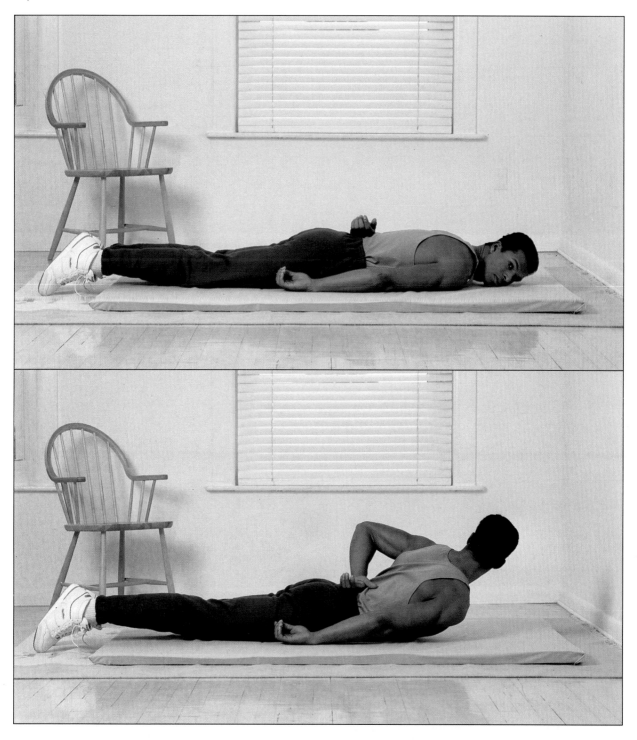

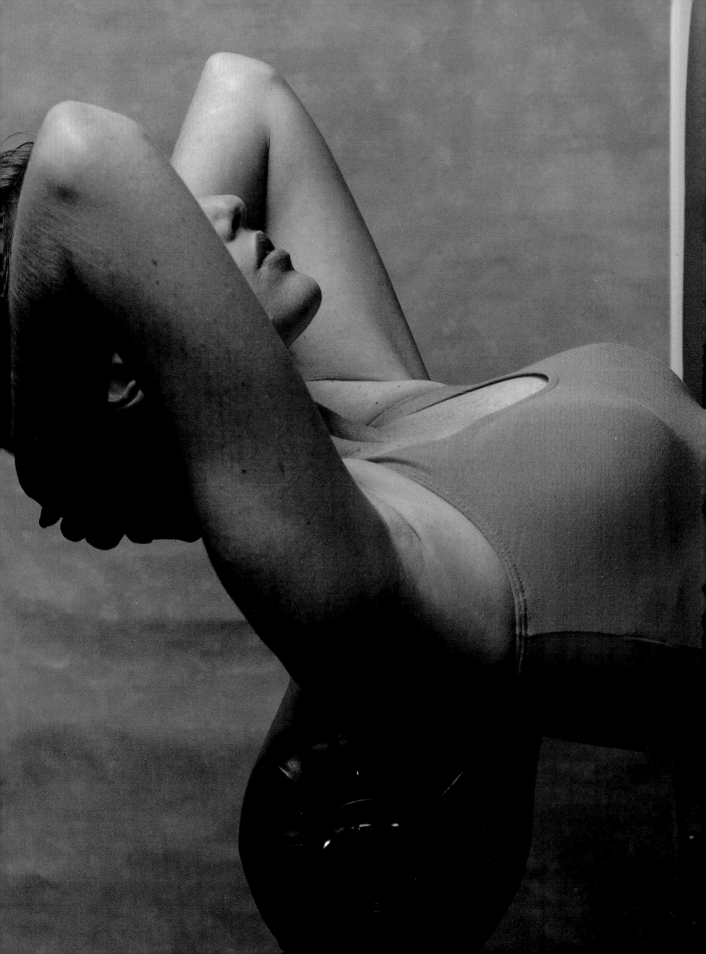

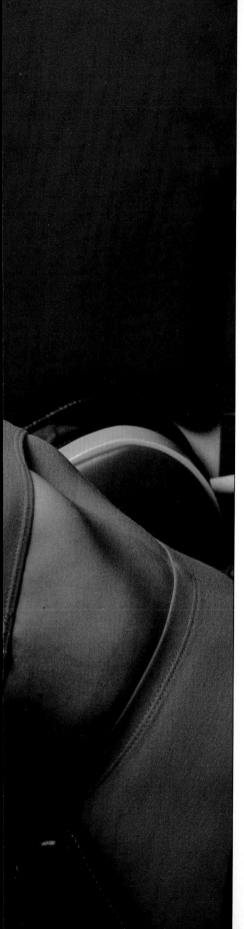

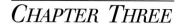
The Machine Workout

Training and shaping muscles with variable resistance

In recent years, many fitness enthusiasts have come to prefer working out in health clubs, commercial gyms and fitness centers. Such establishments have grown in number — there are an estimated 6,500 in the United States — as well as in the kinds of facilities they provide. Of course, going to a club or gym cannot match the convenience of exercising at home, but a club is likely to have machines that are too bulky or expensive for most homes. Machines to build strength come in a variety of sizes and designs, and new models appear constantly. At many health clubs, though, the most popular machines are likely to be referred to as variable resistance machines. These include machines made by Nautilus, the most widely recognized maker, and similar machines from other manufacturers.

Because muscles and bones function as levers, a given weight on a barbell or dumbbell may feel lighter in one position and heavier in another position. The position in which a weight feels heaviest is called the sticking point. In order to exercise a muscle through its full range of motion with free weights, you need to select a weight that is light enough for you to move it through its sticking point. By doing so, however, the muscle is stressed with less than maximum resistance through its range of motion, and your strength gains may take longer. Variable resistance machines have been designed to compensate automatically for a muscle's changes in strength by utilizing cams or levers to vary the resistance, keeping it at maximum throughout the full range of motion *(see box opposite)*. Furthermore, by maintaining your body in a particular position and by making you move a weight along a predetermined path, the machines apply resistance directly to the muscle being worked, isolating that muscle more efficiently than is usually possible with free weights.

Whether training on variable resistance machines develops strength faster or to a greater degree than working with free weights has yet to be established. Both methods of training have produced positive results, and it may be that certain machines are more efficient than others, which may also be true of certain barbell exercises; however, machines do offer some advantages. For people beginning a weight-training program, machines are usually easier to work with and safer to use than free weights. This is because the machines are designed to utilize weighted plates held in place by pins that slide back and forth along a fixed path. You adjust the amount of weight for an exercise simply by inserting a pin at a particular point in the weight stack, rather than by having to load and unload weights onto a barbell. This frees you from worrying about dropping a weight or maintaining your balance during an exercise. The use of pins also allows you to move quickly from machine to machine, so that you can complete your workout in 20 to 30 minutes.

Some advocates of machine training have claimed that, because machines are highly efficient, you can get the best workout by performing only one set of each exercise. However, this single set should be intense enough to achieve momentary muscular failure on the last repetition. In other words, at the end of the set, your muscles should be so fatigued that they cannot move the weight through another repetition. To work this intensely, you will need to experiment over several sessions to find the right amount of weight you need on each machine. But you will find that working to muscular failure can be difficult and even painful. Therefore, you may wish to take more time and perform two or three sets at 80 or 90 percent of your maximum ability.

If you are interested in using machines at a gym or health club, make sure that there is a sufficient variety to give you a full workout. You should be able to perform four to six exercises for the lower body and six to eight for the upper body. Machines should be arranged so that you can work larger muscles before smaller ones, since this is the desirable sequence for the most efficient workout. Your gains in strength will be greatest if you rest a few minutes between machines.

Variable Resistance

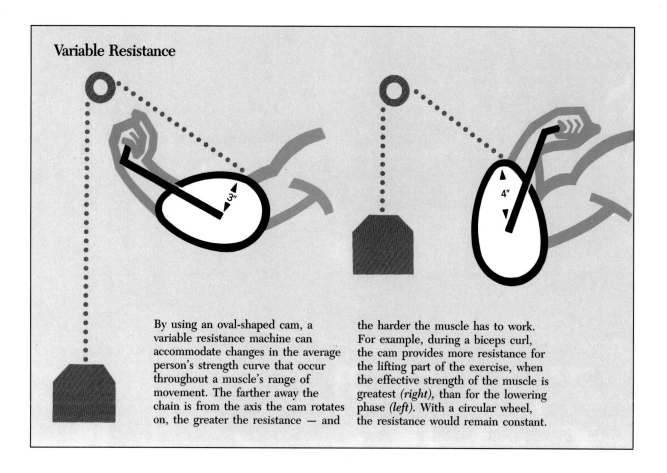

By using an oval-shaped cam, a variable resistance machine can accommodate changes in the average person's strength curve that occur throughout a muscle's range of movement. The farther away the chain is from the axis the cam rotates on, the greater the resistance — and the harder the muscle has to work. For example, during a biceps curl, the cam provides more resistance for the lifting part of the exercise, when the effective strength of the muscle is greatest *(right)*, than for the lowering phase *(left)*. With a circular wheel, the resistance would remain constant.

By moving quickly, you may elevate your heart rate, but this kind of circuit training will not provide you with any true aerobic or endurance benefits.

The workout shown on the following pages is primarily on Nautilus machines, but many exercises on other brands of machines are similar. It is a good idea to have a trainer at your club show you how to adjust any machine you use to suit your height and physique. Keep in mind that, while a machine steers you through the movement of an exercise, you must still observe good form to get the maximum benefit from this type of equipment.

As with free weights, you will need to experiment to find the proper amount of weight for each exercise. For the first five or six sessions, keep the weight at levels that you can lift comfortably for 12 to 15 repetitions. You can then select a heavier weight load that allows you to reach momentary muscular failure in one set. Or, if you do not wish to work to failure, adjust the weight so that you can perform eight to 12 repetitions, stopping just short of failure, and perform each exercise for two sets.

For beginners and intermediates, three workouts a week on machines are optimal, though many people will derive some benefit from working out twice a week. Be sure to rest at least 48 hours between workouts.

Training Techniques

Start your workout with the five-minute warm-up session outlined on page 22. Begin your machine circuit by conditioning the large muscles of the thighs, using such machines as the one on these two pages, which works the quadriceps and hamstrings. You should then move on to the lower legs (*pages 64-65*) and the upper body.

On each machine, focus on the muscles you are exercising; do not grip the handles tightly, tense your face or contract other unengaged muscles. Be sure to move through the exercise in a deliberate, controlled manner; keep your body aligned and avoid twisting or shifting during the movement. In general, take two seconds to raise a weight and four seconds to lower it, pausing slightly between the two movements. Although on some machines it may take longer to move through the full range of motion, you should always move more slowly through the lowering phase than through the lifting phase. Exhale as you raise the weight; inhale as you lower it.

Sit in the leg extension machine with your back firmly against the base and with a folded towel behind your neck. Fasten the belt and place your feet behind the rollers (*below*). **Extend your right leg** (*below right*), **pause briefly and return. Finish with one leg before you work the other.**

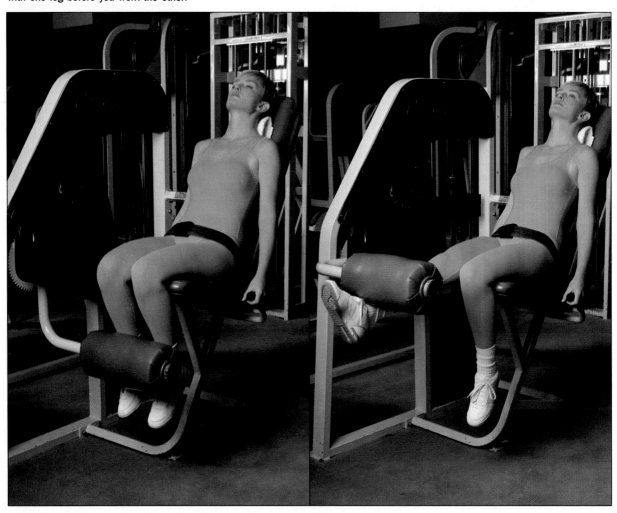

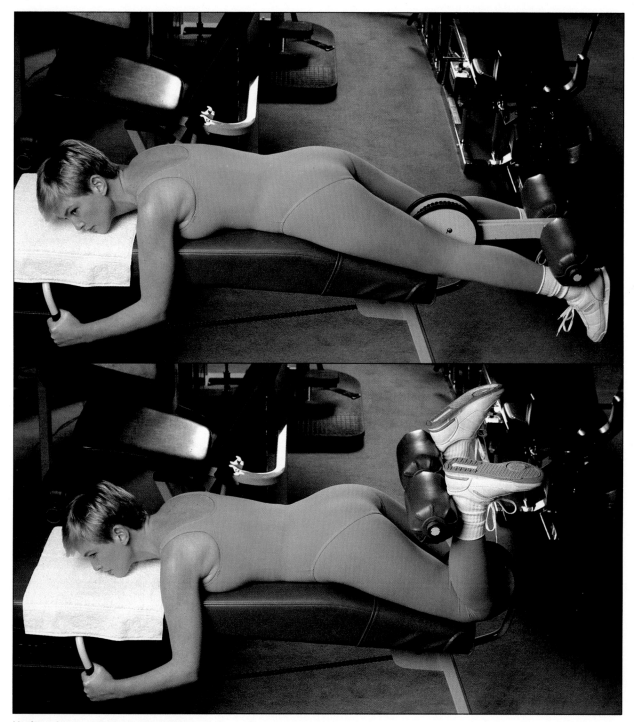

Lie face down on the leg curl machine, slip your feet under the rollers and grasp the handles lightly *(top)*. Draw the rollers toward your buttocks without raising your hips more than one or two inches *(above)*. Pause briefly and return.

61

Abductor and Adductor

To work your outer thighs, sit down in
the abductor machine, place a folded
towel behind your neck and lightly grasp
the handles *(below)*. Using your thighs,
not your ankles, press outward against
the machine *(below right)*. Pause briefly
and return to the starting position.

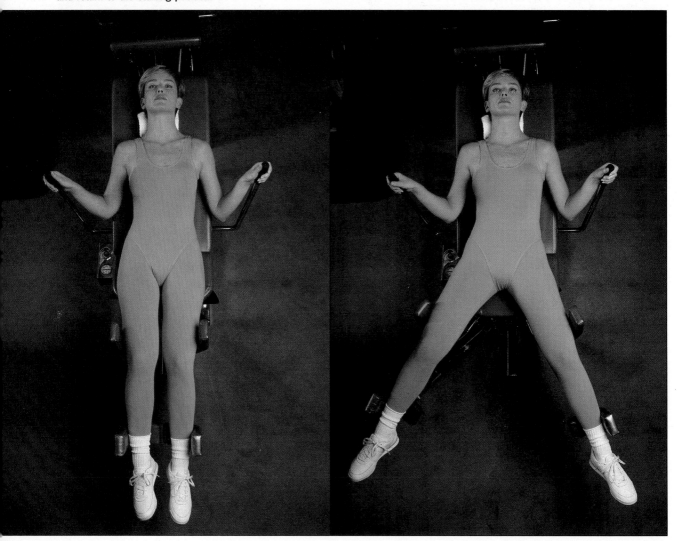

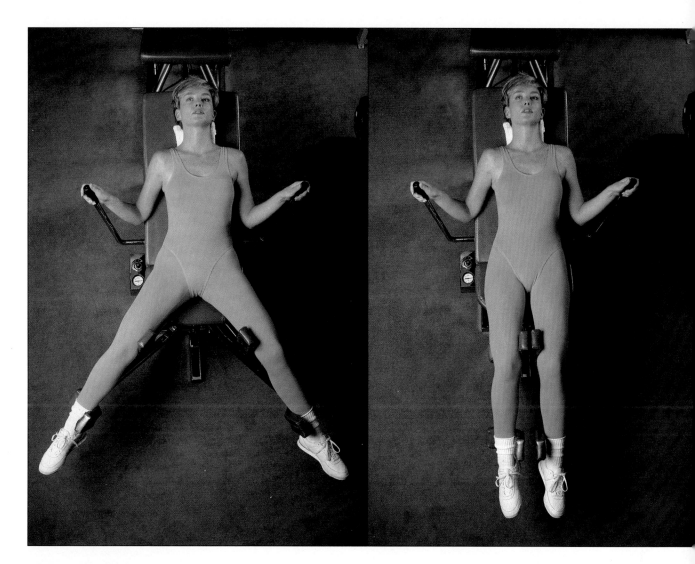

Sit in the adductor machine — which
works the inner thighs — with a towel
behind your neck (above). Squeeze your
legs together, using only the force of your
thigh muscles to resist the force of the
machine (above right). Pause briefly and
return to the starting position.

Multi-Exercise

To condition your calf muscles, attach the hip belt to the multi-exercise machine and adjust it around your waist. Grasp the handles and step onto the platform with the balls of your feet so that your heels drop *(right)*. Rise up on your toes as high as you can without leaning forward or backward *(inset)*. Hold for a second and return. Perform 15 to 20 repetitions of this exercise.

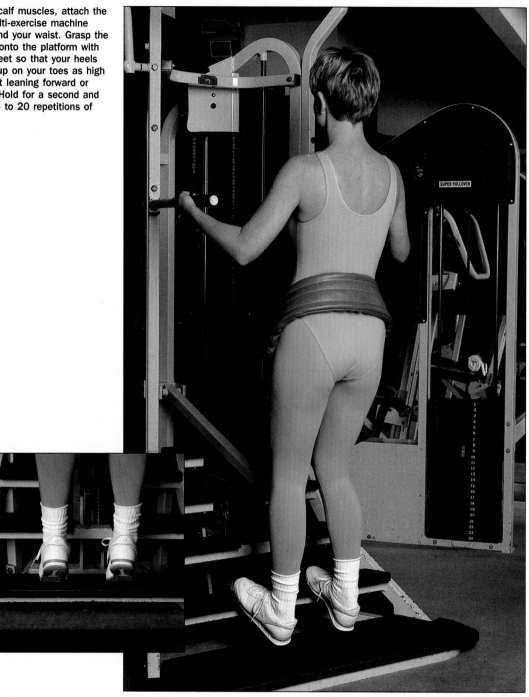

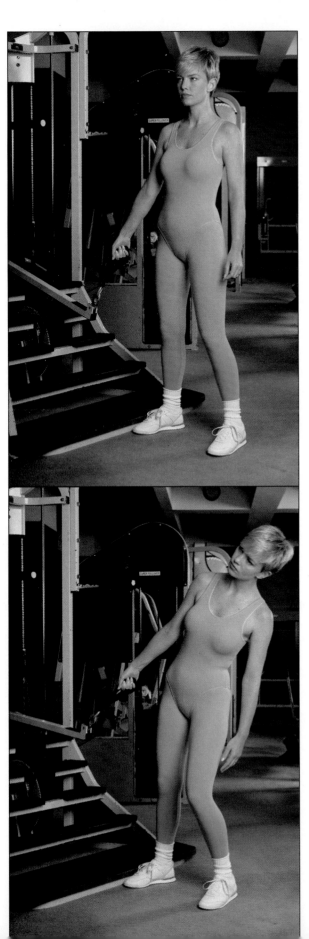

To work the oblique muscles in your sides, attach a hand grip to the multi-exercise machine. Hold the grip in your right hand and stand with your right side facing the machine, your feet about 12 inches apart *(left)*. Keep your right knee straight, bend your left knee and pull away with your body *(below left)*. Return to the starting position. Perform about 15 to 20 repetitions.

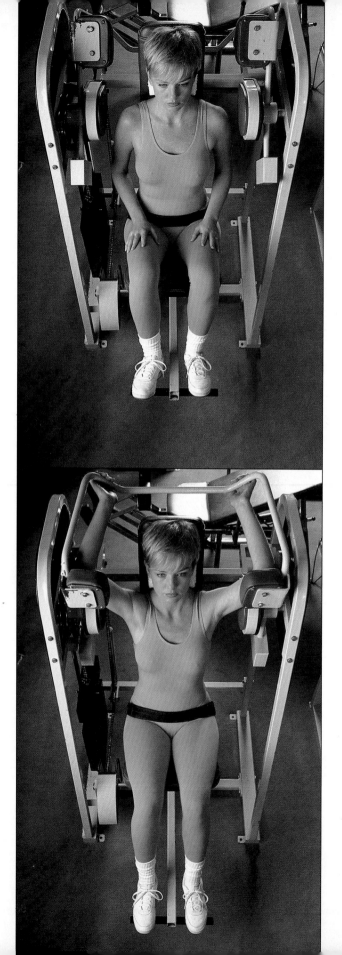

Lat Pull-Over

Sit in the lat pull-over machine, which conditions the latissimus dorsi muscles in your back. Tighten the belt and bring the crossbar into position by depressing the footplate *(left)*. Raise your arms over your head, place your elbows in the pads and rest your fingers lightly on the cross-bar *(below left)*. Release the footplate and slowly draw the crossbar down *(inset opposite)*. Be sure to push with your elbows, not your hands, as you draw the crossbar to your waist *(opposite)*. Pause briefly and return to the starting position.

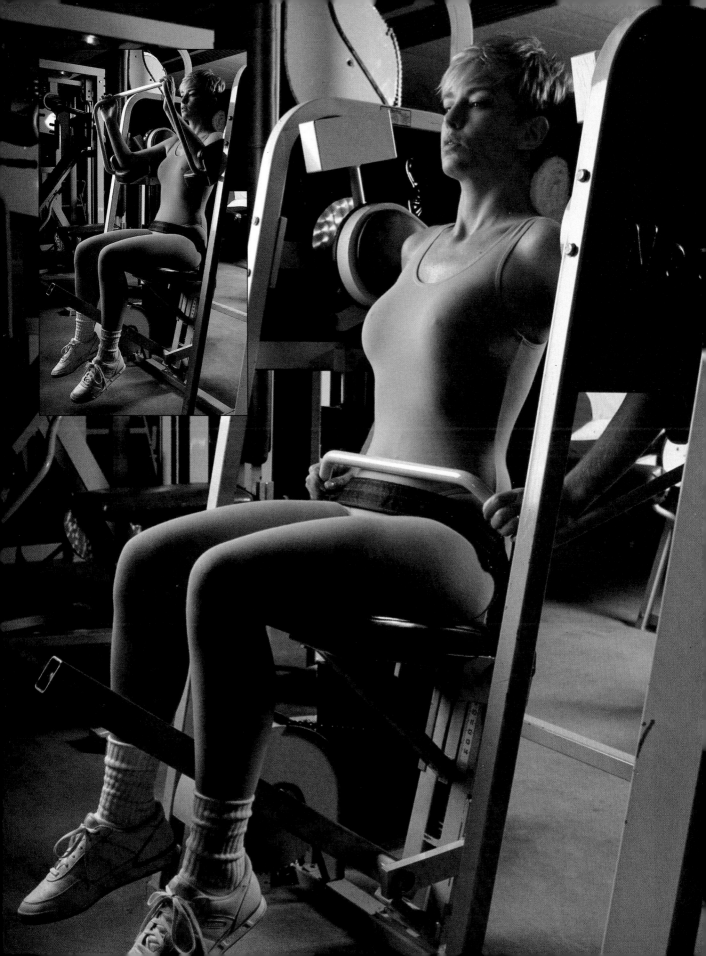

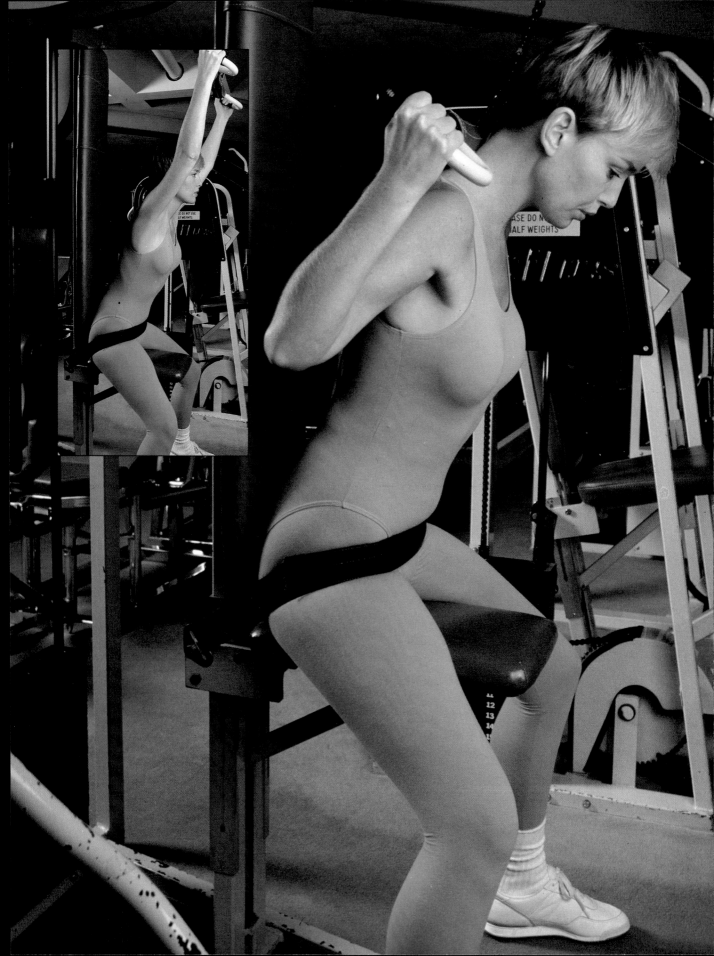

Lat Pull-Down

Sit in the lat pull-down machine and fasten the belt. Reach up and pull the bar down, grip the handles and lean forward, keeping your elbows slightly bent *(inset opposite)*. Pull the bar behind your neck *(opposite)*. Pause briefly and return to the starting position.

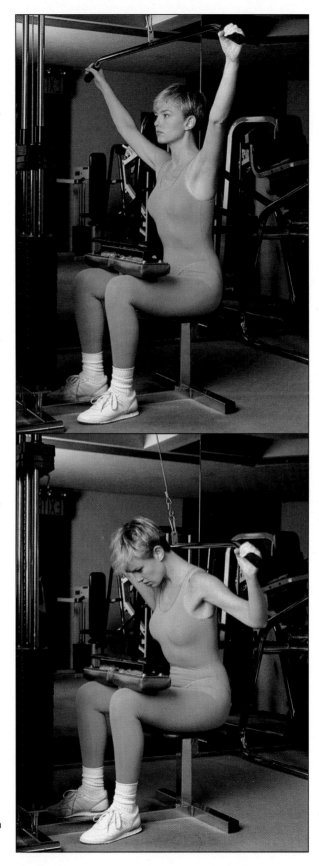

An alternative lat pull-down machine has a padded leg brace to keep you in place. Sit down and slip your legs under the pads so that they hold your lower body firmly on the bench. Reach up and pull down the bar, gripping both handles and keeping your elbows slightly bent *(top right)*. Lean forward and pull the bar down behind your neck *(right)*. Pause briefly and return to the starting position.

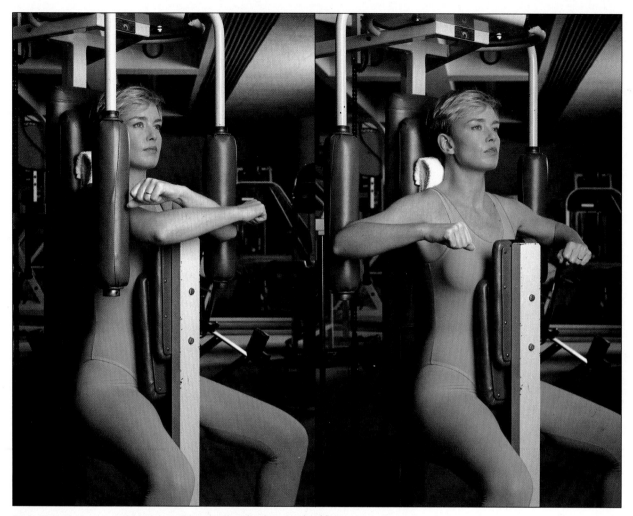

Sit in a rowing torso machine to condition the muscles in your shoulders and upper back. Place your arms through the rollers and cross your forearms *(above left)*. Push back as far as you comfortably can and try to squeeze your shoulder blades together *(above right)*. Pause briefly and return to the starting position.

Rows and Raises

To strengthen the deltoid muscles in your shoulders, sit in a lateral raise machine and fasten the belt. Lightly grip the handle and push out and up with your elbows *(opposite top)*. Raise your elbows until your forearms are parallel to the floor *(opposite)*. Pause briefly and return to the starting position.

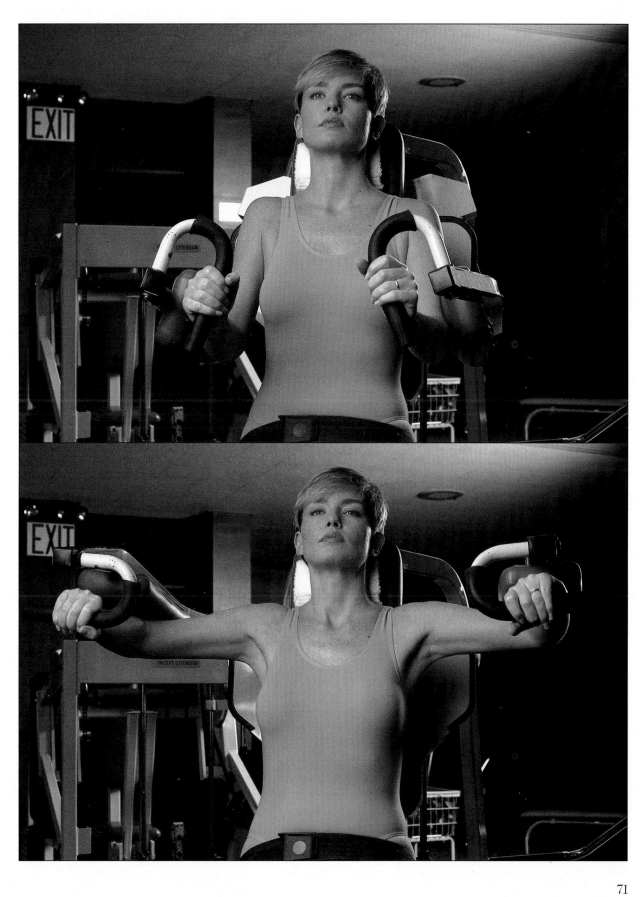

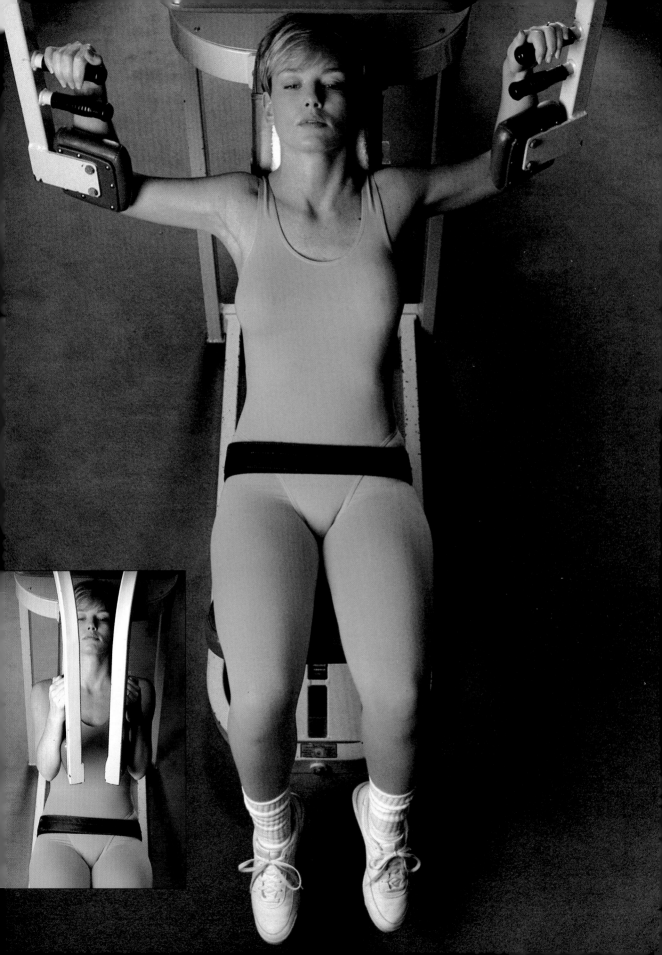

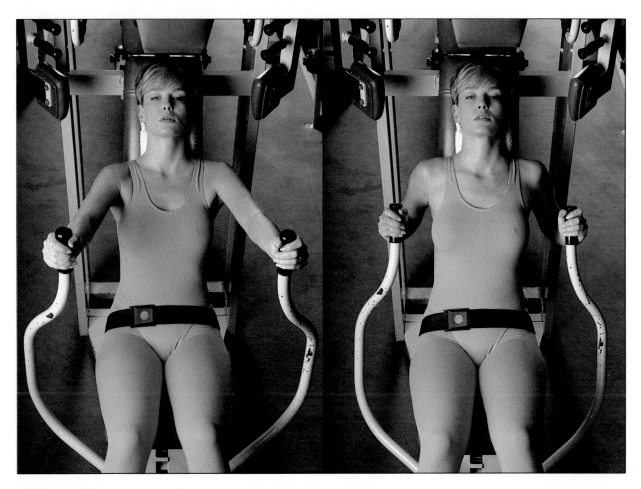

Arm Cross and Decline Press

To strengthen your chest and shoulder
muscles, use the arm-cross machine.
Place a towel behind your neck and
fasten the belt. Place your forearms
against the pads and hold the handles
lightly *(opposite)*. Press with your
forearms toward the center of your chest
(inset). Pause briefly and return to the
starting position. A similar machine offers
both the arm-cross exercise and a decline
press. Complete a set of arm-cross
repetitions first, then perform the decline
press. Place your feet on the footplate
and push the handles into position. Grasp
the handles, release the footplate and
push the handles forward *(above)*. Pause
briefly, then allow the levers to move
back slowly until you feel a stretch in
your chest muscles *(above right)*.

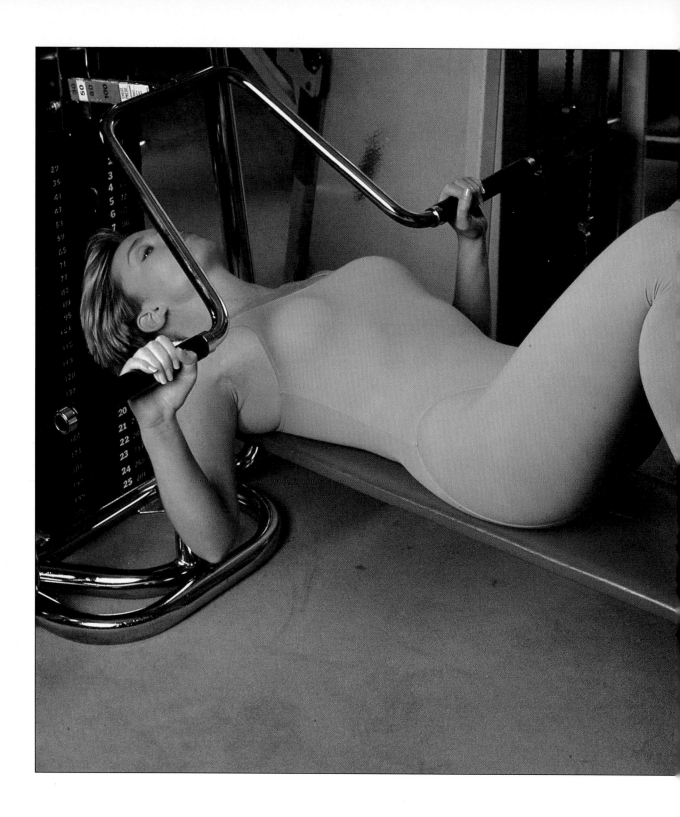

Bench Press

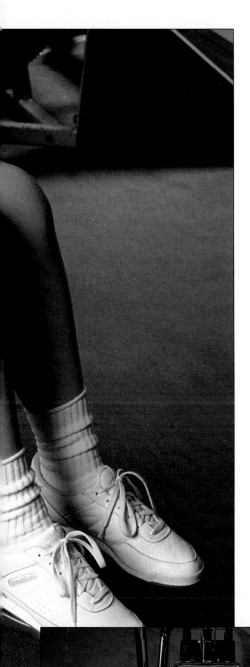

Use a bench-press machine to condition your pectorals, deltoids and triceps; the wider your grip is, the more you will emphasize your pectorals. Lie down with your knees bent and your feet flat on the bench. Place a towel behind your neck and grasp the handles *(left)*. Apply pressure to the handles so that the weights begin to lift off the weight stack *(below left)*. Press the handles up and extend your arms without locking your elbows *(below right)*. Pause briefly and return to the starting position.

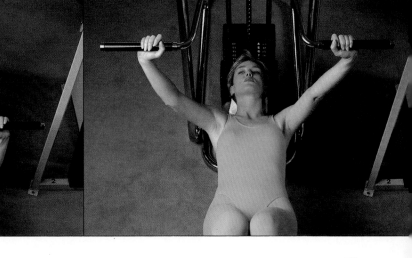

Triceps and Biceps

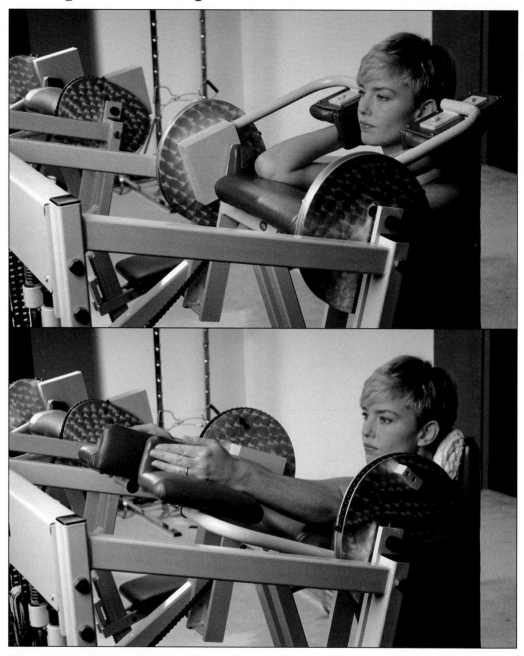

Sit on the triceps machine, place your elbows on the pad and your hands in the grip, palms facing in *(top)*. The seat should be adjusted so that your shoulders are slightly lower than your elbows. Extend your arms together, but do not lock your elbows *(above)*. Pause briefly and return to the starting position.

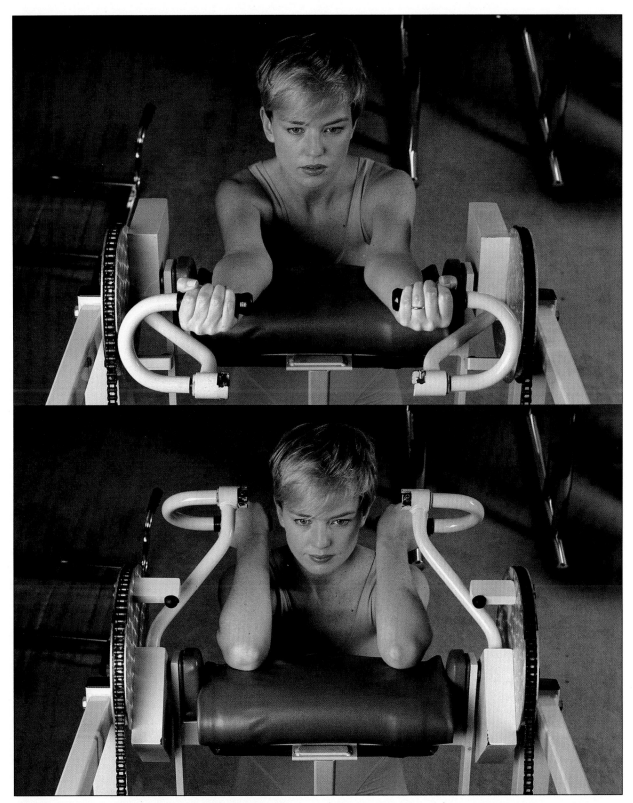

Straddle the biceps machine, place your elbows on the pad, grip the handles and pull them halfway up. Then sit and lower the handles until your elbows are slightly bent *(top)*. Curl the handles back together until your hands just about touch your ears *(above)*. Pause briefly and return to the starting position.

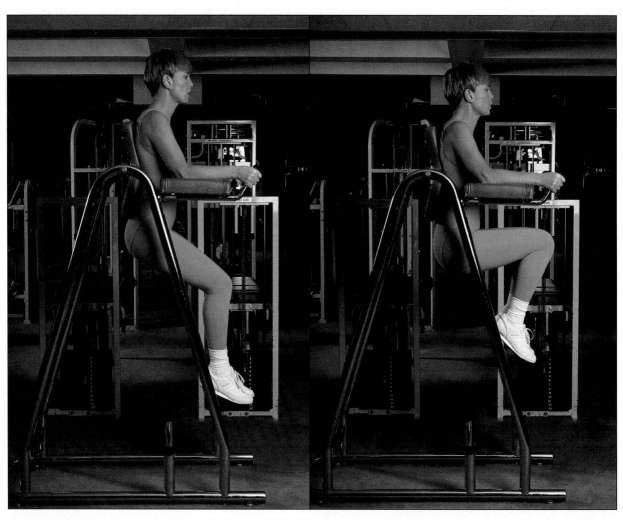

Hip Flexors and
Lower Back

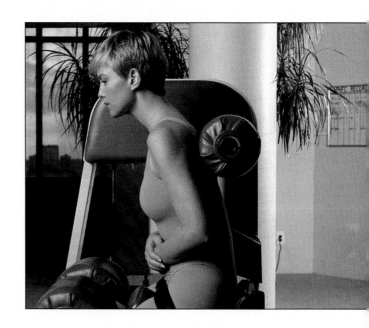

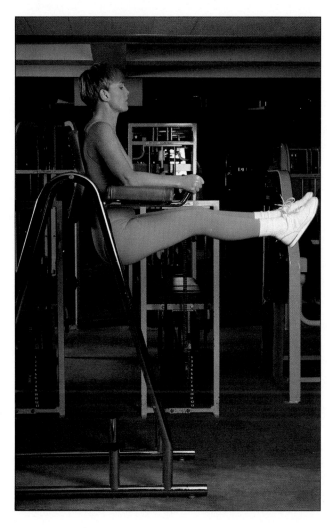

This exercise should be done in conjunction with the abdominal exercises shown on pages 52-53. (If you have had back pain, do not perform this or the exercise below. Stop doing either exercise if it causes any back pain.) Step up in a hip-flexor apparatus, grip the handles, place your forearms on the pads and let your legs dangle. Draw up your knees slightly *(far left)*. Raise your knees so that your thighs are parallel to the floor *(center left)*. Pause briefly and return to the starting position. As an advanced exercise, keep your legs extended with your knees slightly bent. Raise your legs slowly until they are parallel to the floor *(near left)*. Pause briefly and return to the starting position.

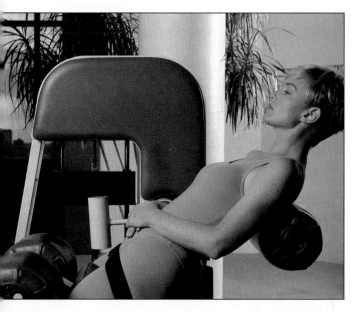

Sit straddling the lower back machine. Place your thighs under the rollers, attach the belt and cross your hands over your abdomen *(far left)*. Push against the pad until your back is straight, at about a 45-degree angle to your lower legs *(left)*. Do not arch your back. Pause briefly and return to the starting position.

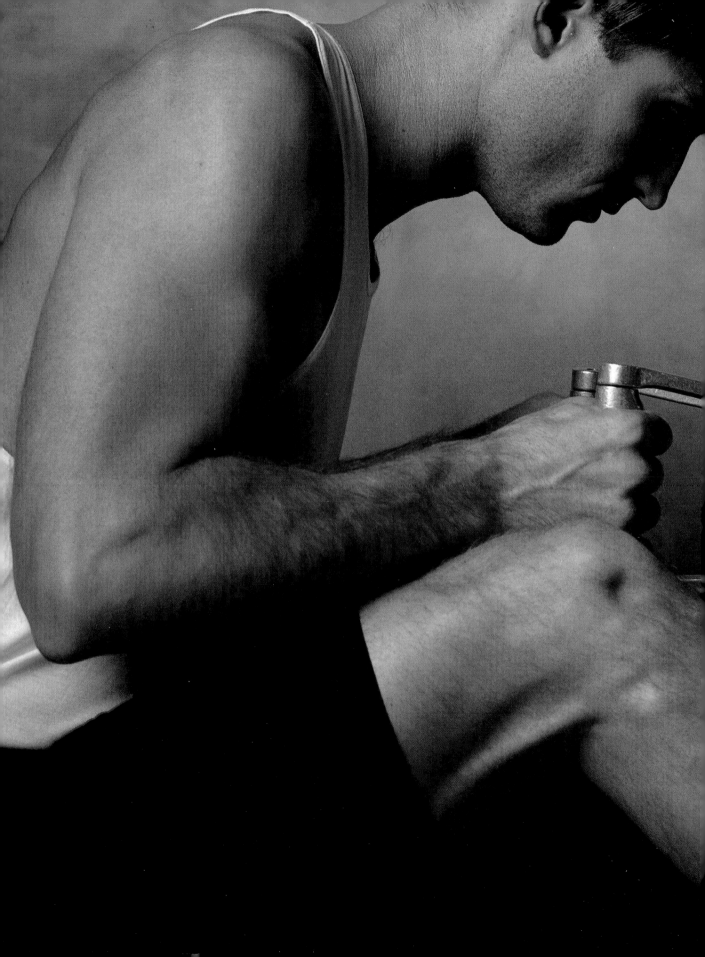

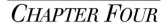

CHAPTER FOUR

Advanced Weight Training

Concentrated free-weight exercises for shaping any of the major muscle groups

Although variable resistance machines are effective tools for building strength and muscle tone, most serious body builders prefer training with barbells, dumbbells and machines that provide the same sort of equal, or isotonic, resistance to a muscle as free weights do. Experienced body builders may use variable resistance machines for isolating and strengthening specific muscles, but their most notable gains in muscle mass are usually accomplished with free weights. The principal reason for this appears to be that free weights allow you not only to target a particular muscle group, but to engage other muscles that assist in the work *(see box page 83)*. Once they are conditioned, these assisting, or synergistic, muscles help you to increase the weight you use in training the target muscles to stimulate the most growth in muscle fibers.

Variable resistance machines, on the other hand, are designed to work target muscles in isolation, without the assistance of surrounding muscles. As a result, you cannot train the target muscle with the same amount of weight as you can with free weights. This synergy principle has generally been supported by research comparing the benefits of free weights and machines, although the differences in strength gains in some studies have been so small that individual training variations may explain them. Still, most body builders maintain that free weights provide the greatest versatility. Machines can also be adjusted only for a certain range of height and physique; weights are appropriate for people of virtually any height or physique. Finally, using free weights can help improve your coordination because you must always control and balance the weights yourself, without the help of the machines.

The exercises in this chapter, which are grouped according to major muscle groups, can be used to shape and build specific body parts. These exercises are not designed as a single routine, but rather to extend — and add variety to — the basic training regimens in the preceding chapters. You should perform the exercises only after you have toned and conditioned your muscles with one of these regimens, which can take beginners from six to 10 weeks.

A number of these more advanced exercises can be performed at home if you have a basic home gym. However, if you are serious about body building or advanced strength training, you should consider a health club or commercial gym. In a well-equipped gym, you will find Olympic barbells, which are about seven feet long and which can be loaded with enough weight — 700 pounds or more — to challenge even the most powerful weight lifter. Most gyms also have leg extension machines, leg curl machines, lat machines and other devices to help you shape your body. A good commercial gym will also offer several types of benches to allow you to adjust your body position so that you can apply the overload of weights effectively to different parts of your body.

An important safety item that you should wear whenever you lift heavy weights is a lifting belt. This wide leather belt, when worn snugly around the waist, helps support your lower back and prevent injuries while you perform such routines as the dead lift on pages 84 and 85 or T-bar rows on page 100. Most gyms provide lifting belts.

When you first perform some of these more advanced exercises, you may be tempted to cheat by using momentum rather than the strength of the muscles. This can place unwanted stress on assisting muscles, joints and ligaments, and it can also throw you off balance; cheating also reduces the stress placed on muscles you want to strengthen. One way to avoid cheating is by performing the exercises in front of a mirror and observing your form. Another technique is to train with a partner, who can point out any lapses in form and even lightly hold your body in position as you lift.

A partner can help you in other ways as well. For most exercises, he or she can assist you in finishing a set, when you may be struggling to push a barbell past the sticking point, or the most difficult position of a repetition, where your leverage is weakest. Standing in front of you

Synergistic Muscles

When you perform lifts with free weights, you train not only the muscles most directly stressed by the weight, but smaller synergistic, or assisting, muscles. For example, lifters perform the exercise at right — a one-arm row — primarily to condition the latissimus dorsi muscles in the back, which act to pull the arms backward. Yet muscles in the arm and shoulder are actively engaged as well.

Free-weight training not only conditions your major muscle groups, but also strengthens the assisting muscles, which help to stabilize your body, support your limbs and maintain your posture during a lift. In this way, weight lifting can improve your physique generally.

In addition, lifting free weights improves your coordination by improving the neuromuscular pathways that connect your muscles to the central nervous system.

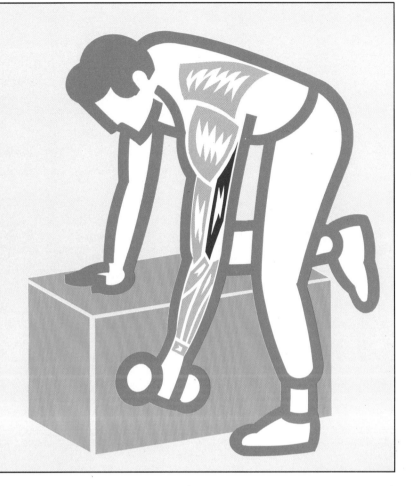

or behind you, depending on the exercise, a partner applies just enough pressure on the bar so that you can complete the repetition smoothly and in strict form while lifting the maximum amount of weight. And should you be in danger of dropping a weight because of fatigue or cramping, your partner can help steady the weight and so prevent what could be a serious injury.

In addition, a partner is necessary for many eccentric training exercises, or negative work, in which you reverse the lifting motion of an exercise and lower a weight while resisting the force of gravity. Because lowering is easier than lifting, an eccentric exercise requires more weight to overload your muscles than does a concentric, or lifting, exercise. Yet you must lift this greater weight to a starting position, as in the negative leg curl on page 91, and you can accomplish this with the help of a training partner.

Usually, the best place to find the type of equipment used in the following exercises is a commercial training facility. When comparing gyms, look at cleanliness, neatness and the condition of the equipment. Exercise stations should not be crowded together: Most weight-room accidents occur when lifters get in each other's way.

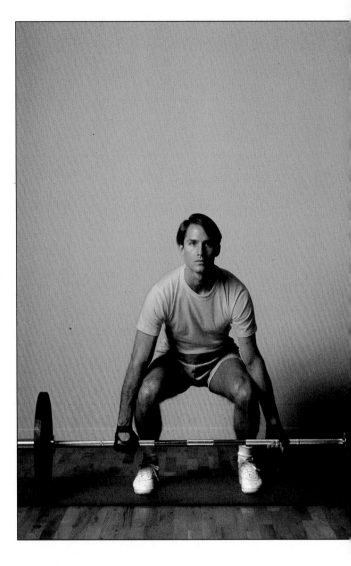

Thighs/1

The pleasing sculpted look you can achieve when you condition your thighs seems to occur quickly, compared to the time it takes to shape other muscles. However, this is due to the size of the thigh muscles — the largest in the body — rather than any difference between the upper leg muscles and other muscle groups.

Chief among the muscles in the region are the quadriceps, along the front of the thigh, and the hamstrings, along the back of the thigh. The four quadriceps muscles collectively extend the knee and stabilize the kneecap. When you sit on a leg extension machine and lift your legs, as on page 88, you are using the quadriceps. The opposing ham-

strings flex the knee or draw your lower leg back. Other muscles in the thigh region that the exercises on these two pages and the following six will develop include the hip flexors, which bend your trunk and lift your thigh, and the hip extensors, which pull your thigh back when you are standing. Be sure to perform these exercises for both sides of your body.

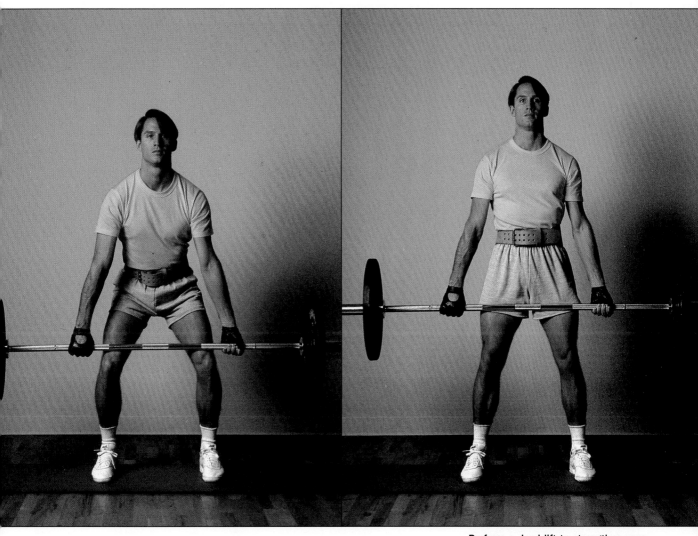

Perform a dead lift to strengthen your quadriceps, lower back and buttocks. Place a barbell on the floor and spread your feet about 16 to 20 inches apart. Bend down and grip the bar with your hands just outside your knees, one palm facing toward you, the other away *(left)*. Keeping your head up and your back straight, lift the bar while you exhale *(center)*. Stand erect but do not lock your knees *(above)*. Return to the starting position, inhaling on your way down.

Thighs/2

Step-ups with a dumbbell are another excellent quadriceps-shaping exercise. Hold the dumbbell in your right hand at your side. Stand in front of an exercise bench and place your right foot on the bench *(inset)*. Keeping your left foot off the bench, step up *(right)*, then return to the starting position.

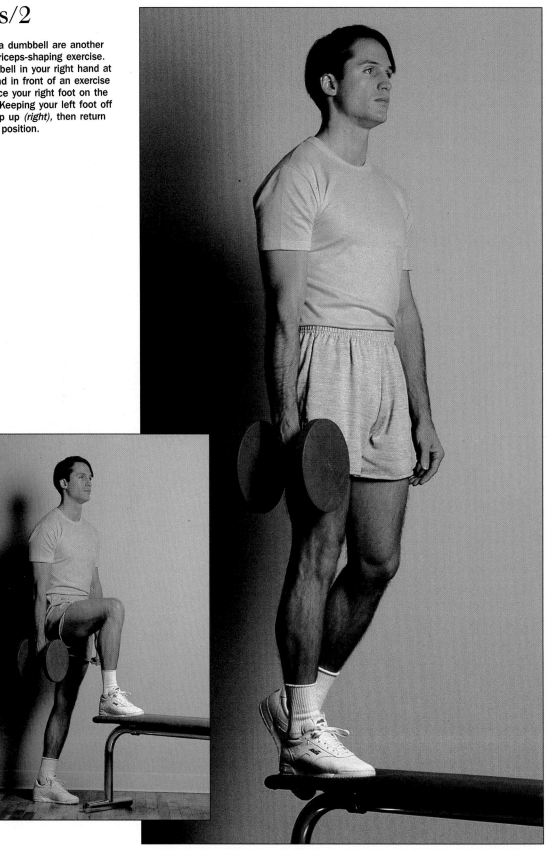

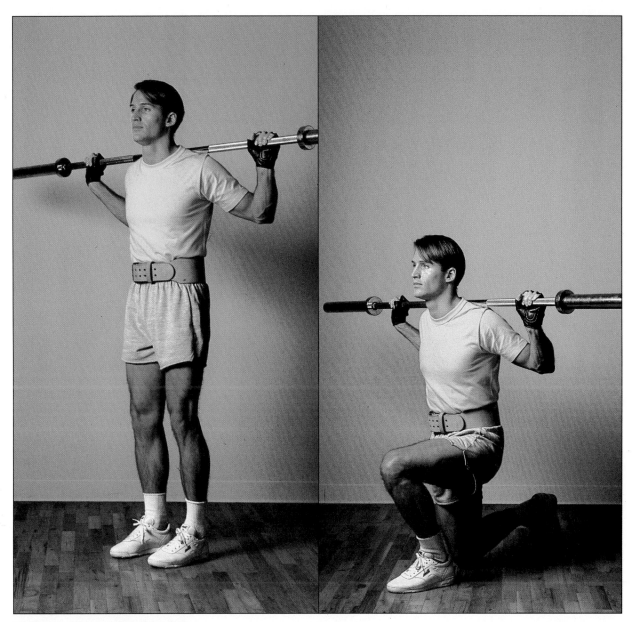

The front lunge is popular among body builders for working the quadriceps and gluteals. Place a barbell across your upper back. Keep your back straight, head up, feet apart and knees slightly bent *(above)*. Take a step forward with your left foot and drop your right knee to within an inch of the floor *(above right)*, as you did for the lunge on page 34. Return to the starting position.

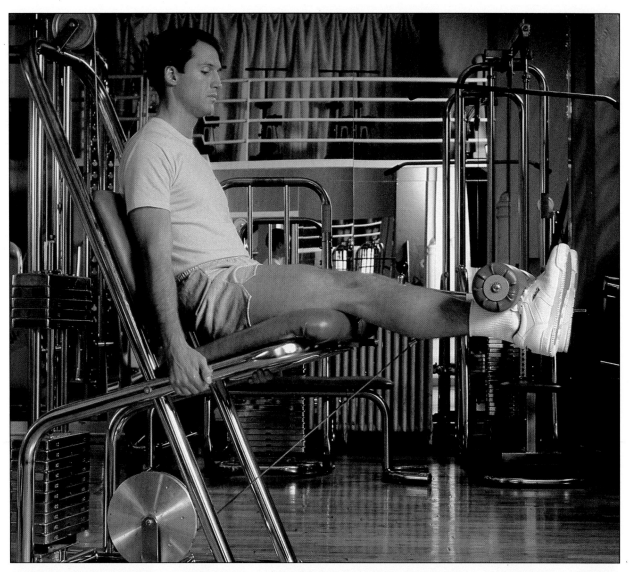

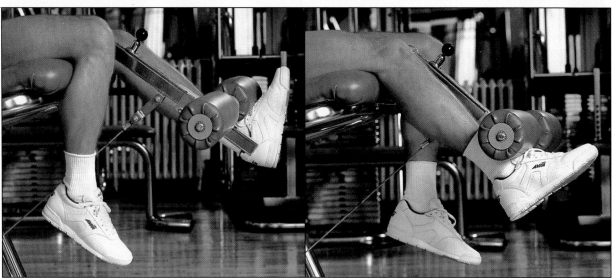

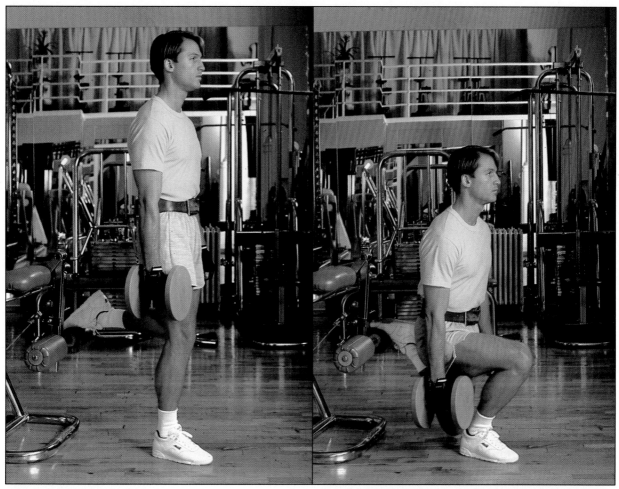

Thighs/3

A more intense version of the lunge on page 87, the one-leg squat, is performed holding a dumbbell at your side in each hand. Bend your left knee and place your foot on a bench behind you *(above left)*. Then drop your left knee and bend your right knee until your right thigh is parallel to the floor *(above)*. Be sure to keep your shoulders back and your head up. Push up and return to the starting position.

Leg extensions isolate the quadriceps, and negative accentuated leg extensions — in which you lift enough weight to tax both legs, then lower that weight with only one leg — provide an even greater stimulus. Sit in a leg extension machine and fasten the belt around your waist. Place your feet under both rollers and extend them together *(opposite top)*. Relax your right leg so that only your left leg is extended and supports the rollers *(far left)*. Then slowly lower your left foot. Repeat the exercise by extending both feet, but this time let the left foot drop, then lower your right foot *(near left)*.

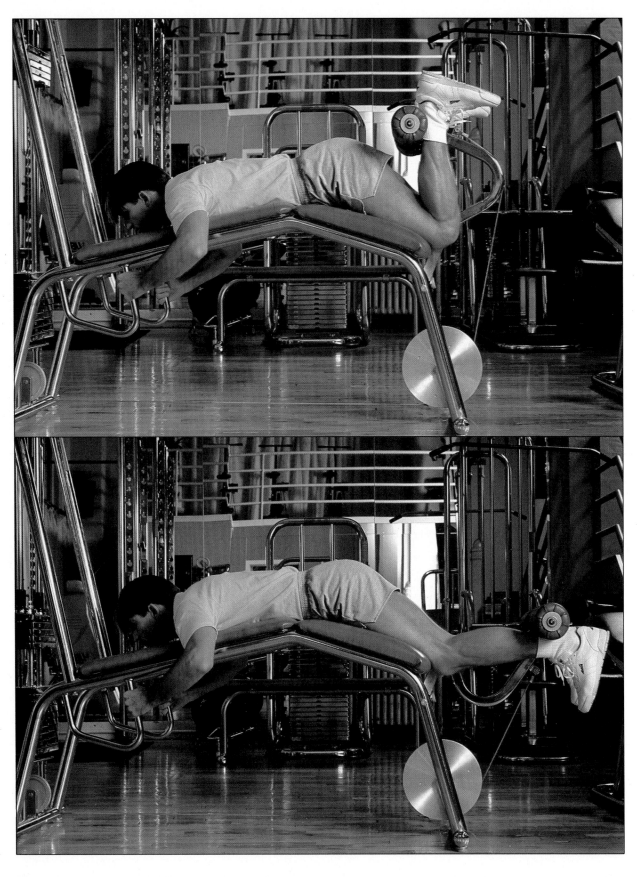

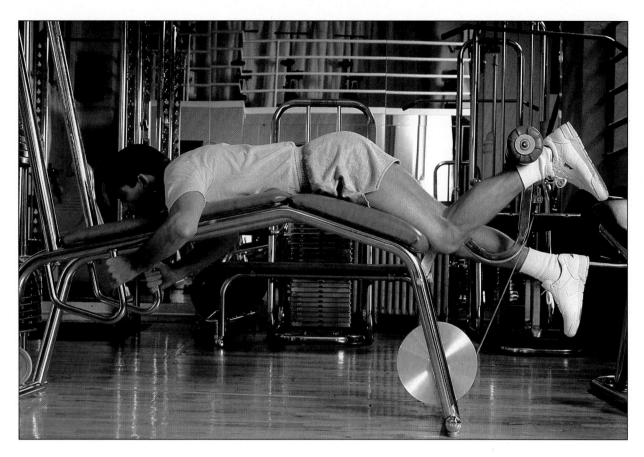

Thighs/4

Perform negative accentuated leg curls
to condition your hamstrings. Raise the
rollers with both feet until your lower
legs are perpendicular to the floor.
Drop your right foot and lower your
left slowly *(above)*.

An alternative to the exercise above is
the negative curl, for which you need a
partner. Lie face down on a leg curl
machine with both feet under rollers that
have been loaded with slightly more
weight than you can raise on your own.
Your partner should stand beside the
machine and help you pull up the rollers
until your lower legs are perpendicular
to the floor *(opposite above)*. On your
own, let the rollers down slowly, keeping
your feet together *(opposite)*.

Calves

Your calf muscles act to pull your heel up and extend your foot. When conditioned, they help you maintain your balance and provide an appealing shape to your entire leg. The primary muscles of the calves, the gastrocnemius and the soleus, constitute a powerful muscle mass that extends down the back of your lower leg and attaches to your Achilles tendon.

Because of their density, trained calf muscles will not tire easily, so for the exercises here you can perform more repetitions than for most other muscles — 20 to 40 repetitions for each set rather than the standard 10 to 15 per set.

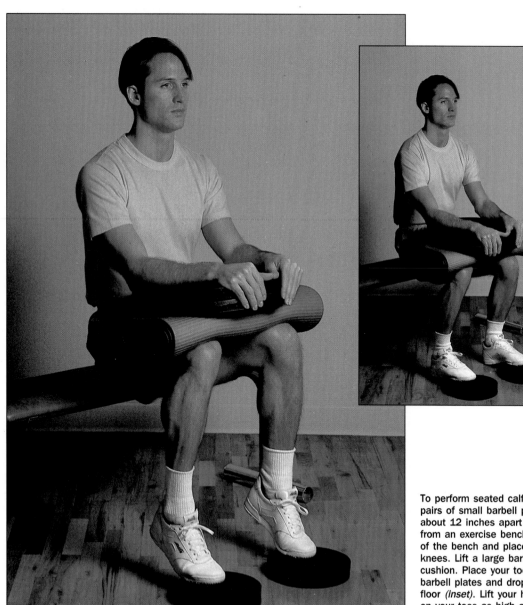

To perform seated calf raises, place two pairs of small barbell plates on the floor about 12 inches apart and 12 inches from an exercise bench. Sit on the edge of the bench and place a cushion on your knees. Lift a large barbell plate onto the cushion. Place your toes on the small barbell plates and drop your heels to the floor *(inset)*. Lift your heels and rise up on your toes as high as possible *(left)*. Return to the starting position.

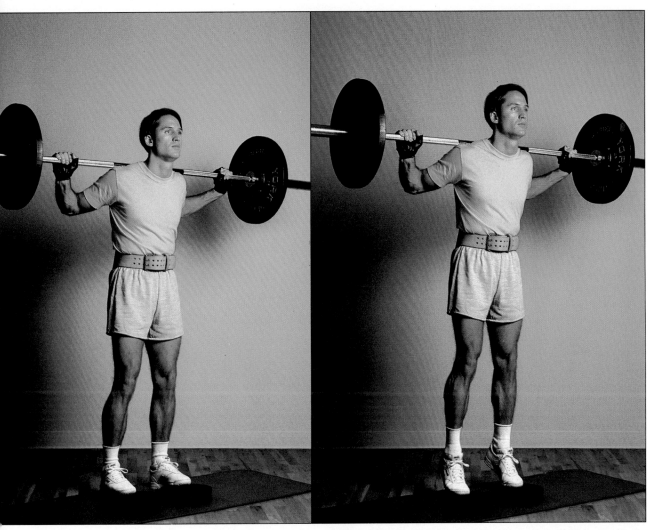

Perform standing barbell calf raises as an advanced alternative to the seated version. Place two pairs of small barbell plates on the floor about 12 inches apart. Lift a barbell onto your upper back and place your toes and the balls of your feet on the small barbell plates. Let your heels rest on the floor *(above left)*. Lift your heels off the floor and rise up on your toes as high as possible *(above)*. Return to the starting position.

Shoulders/1

Gym work to strengthen your primary shoulder muscles — the deltoid and upper trapezius — will give you the appearance of having broader shoulders. Concentrating effort in this area should strengthen your upper back and neck, which will contribute to improved posture.

The deltoid, a large triangular muscle that originates on the collarbone and shoulder blade, and passes over the shoulder joint, gives the shoulder its rounded appearance. The principal action of the deltoid is to raise the arm straight outward. It can also draw the arm forward or backward. In fact, the deltoid is involved in all arm movements; therefore, virtually any arm exercise will work the deltoid to some extent.

The trapezius originates at the base of the skull and along the upper spinal column and extends to the collarbone and shoulder blade. You can effectively condition the trapezius by holding dumbbells or a weighted barbell while standing and performing shoulder shrugs. Other exercises for the deltoid and the trapezius are shown on these two pages and the following two.

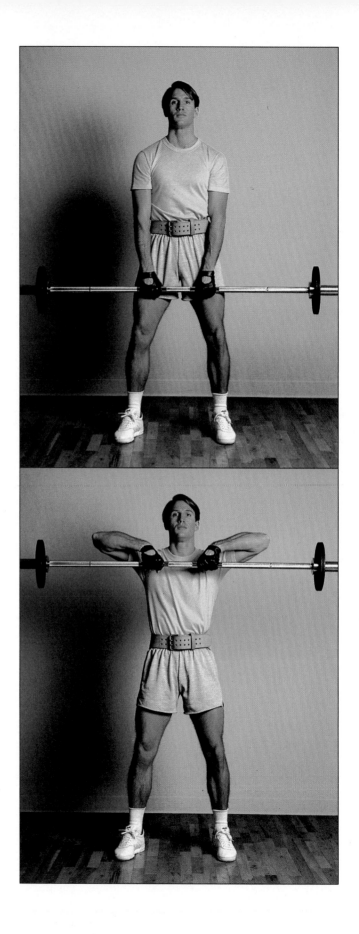

Perform upright rows to strengthen your deltoids. Stand erect with your feet apart and your knees slightly bent. Grasp a weighted barbell with your hands about 12 inches apart and your palms facing in *(top right)*. Lift the bar straight up from the elbows until it is just under your chin *(right)*. Return to the starting position.

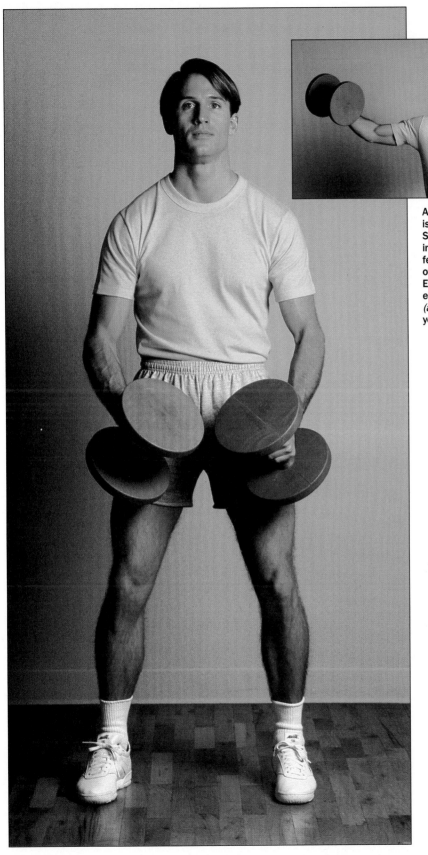

A good exercise for the middle deltoids is the side lateral raise with bent arms. Stand in a quarter-squat position bending forward slightly at the waist with your feet apart and knees flexed. Hold a pair of dumbbells near your upper thighs *(left)*. Extend your arms sideways, bringing your elbows up and lifting your whole body *(above)*. Do not raise the dumbbells above your head.

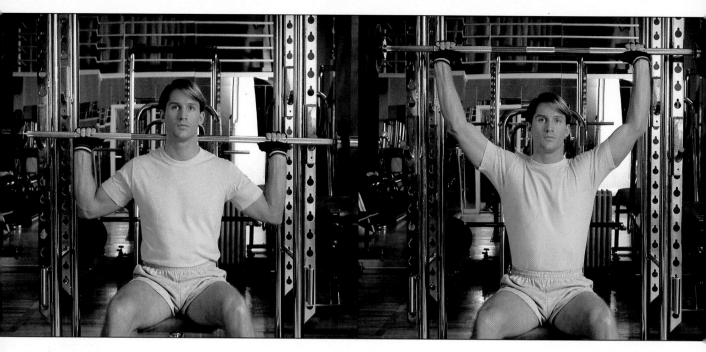

Shoulders/2

Sit erect on a bench while holding a
barbell behind your neck to perform a
seated military press *(above)*. Press the
barbell upward until your elbows are
almost fully extended, being sure to
tighten your abdominals, and keep
your back straight *(above right)*. Return
to the starting position.

Lie on an incline bench and hold a
weighted barbell with a wide grip about
an inch off your chest *(top right)*. Extend
your arms and press straight upward but
do not lock your elbows *(right)*. Return to
the starting position.

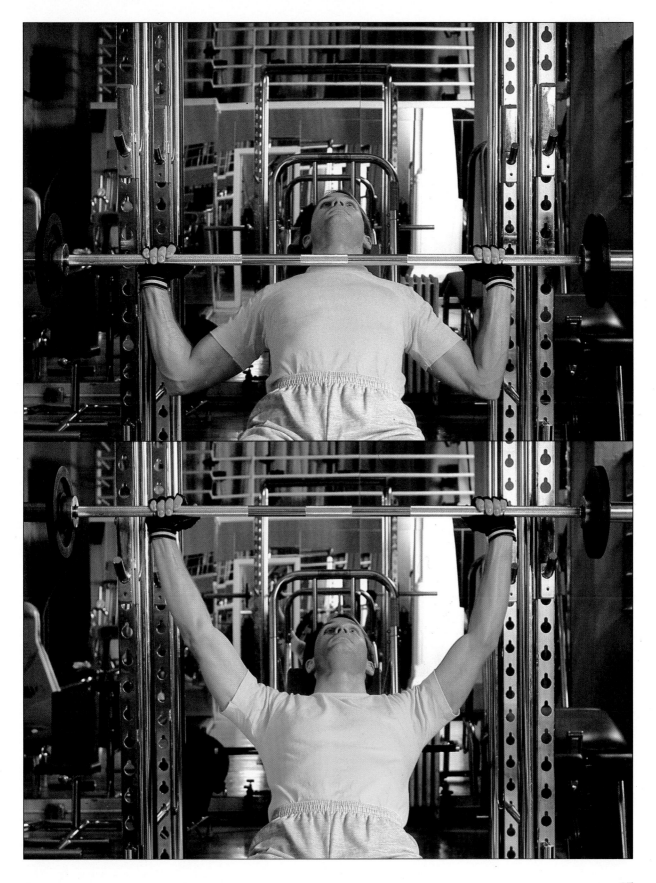

Lats/1

Body builders work to achieve the desired V-shaped back muscle definition by exercising to develop the latissimus dorsi. Commonly called lats, these broad muscles originate along the lower half of your spinal column, reaching the top of your hipbone. The lats fan out to form the back of your armpits. These muscles work to pull your arms in behind your back.

Body building gyms almost always have apparatus to help condition your lats. The equipment may include pulleys and lat pull-down machines, as well as barbells. Two of the most powerful lat developers using this type of equipment are the pulley pull and the T-bar row, shown on this and the following pages. For maximal intensity, a lat pull-down should be performed with a wide-grip on the bar and a pull-down to the chest — not, as widely believed, behind the head.

Sit in front of the pulley machine and place your feet against the footrests. Keeping your knees and elbows slightly bent, reach forward, grasp the pulley handles and apply enough tension to lift the weights slightly off the weight stack *(inset)*. Then pull the handles directly back to the sides of your chest *(right)*. Return to the starting position. Retain control of the weights at all times so that you do not let the weight stack crash at the extended position.

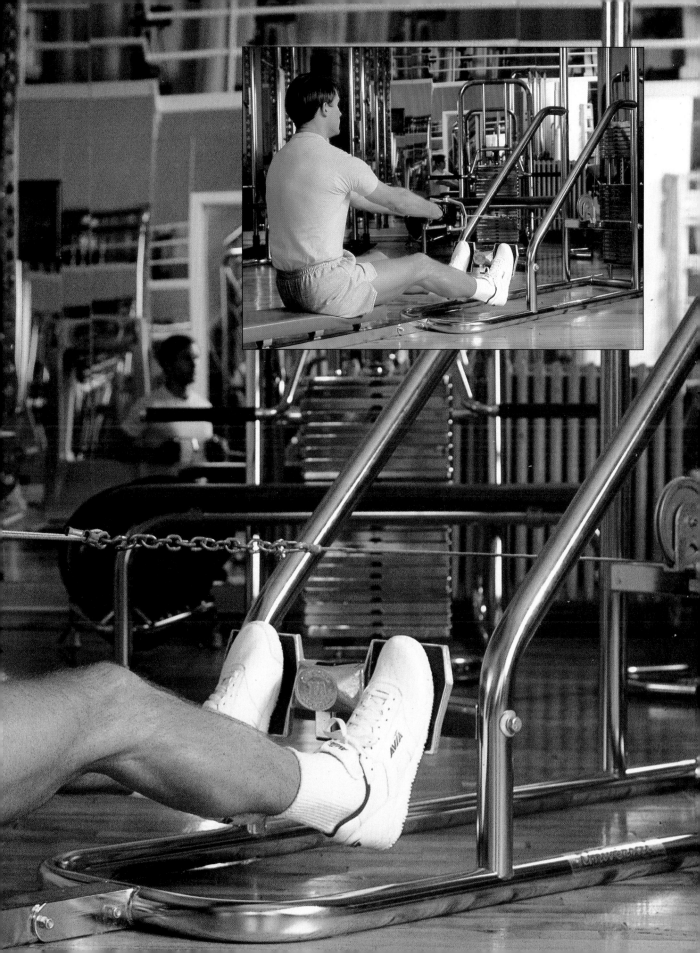

Lats/2

T-bar rows are ideal for conditioning your upper back, particularly the lats. Secure one end of an empty barbell at the corner of a room or against an immovable object and then place weights on the other end. Straddle the bar and face the weighted end, gripping it just below the weight. Pull the bar up off the floor but keep your knees flexed and your elbows slightly bent *(right)*. Then pull the bar up, keeping your elbows in, until the weights touch your chest *(below right)*. Return to the starting position.

Sit down at a lat pull-down machine, fasten yourself in and reach up to grasp the bar. Pull the bar so that the weights you are lifting are just above the weight stack and your elbows are slightly bent *(inset opposite)*. Pull the bar straight down to your chest *(opposite)*. Return to the starting position.

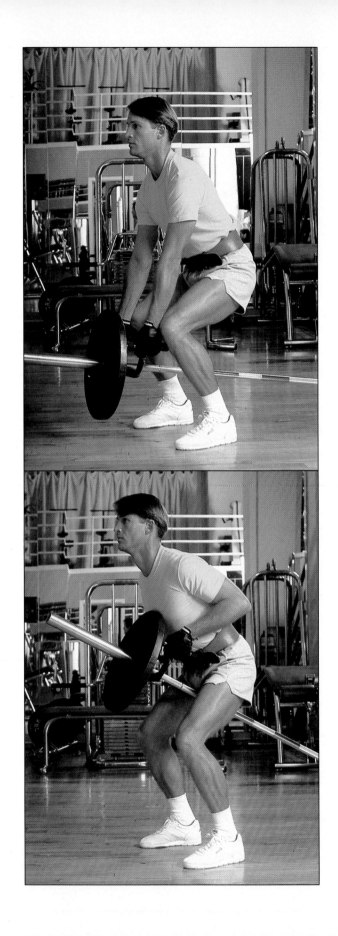

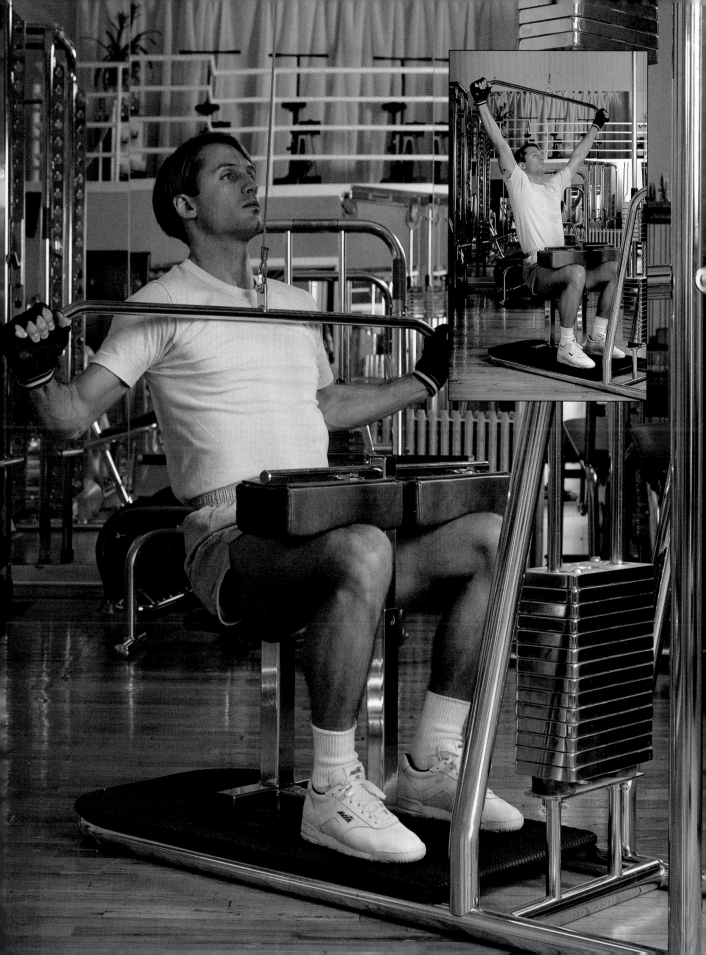

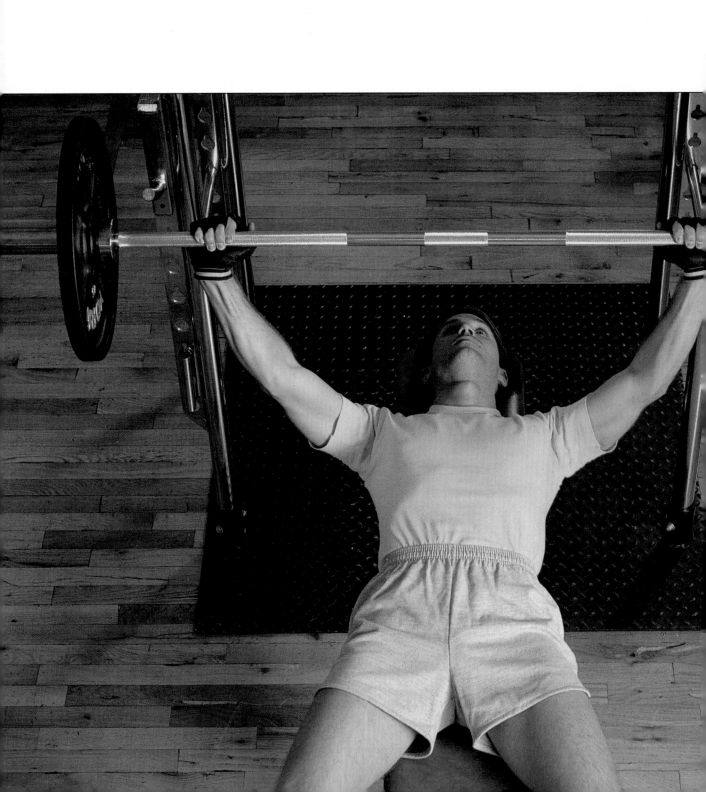

Chest/1

A muscular chest has long been considered a sign of strength. Professional body builders, for instance, pay particular attention to the development of their chest muscles.

Commonly called the pecs, the pectoralis major muscles of the chest swing your arms forward to draw them across your chest, as you do when you throw a ball. In addition, pecs can pull out and expand the chest.

The exercises shown here and on the following two pages — the wide-grip bench press, the decline dumbbell fly and the flat fly — all stress the pectoral muscles maximally.

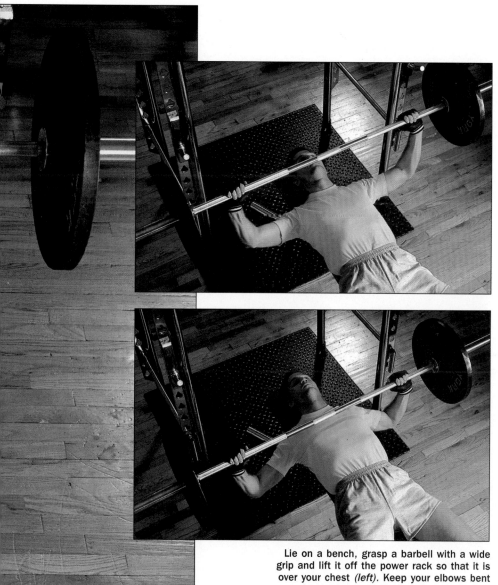

Lie on a bench, grasp a barbell with a wide grip and lift it off the power rack so that it is over your chest *(left)*. Keep your elbows bent and turned out, slowly lowering the barbell without arching your back *(top)* until the bar is about one inch off your chest *(above)*. Return to the starting position.

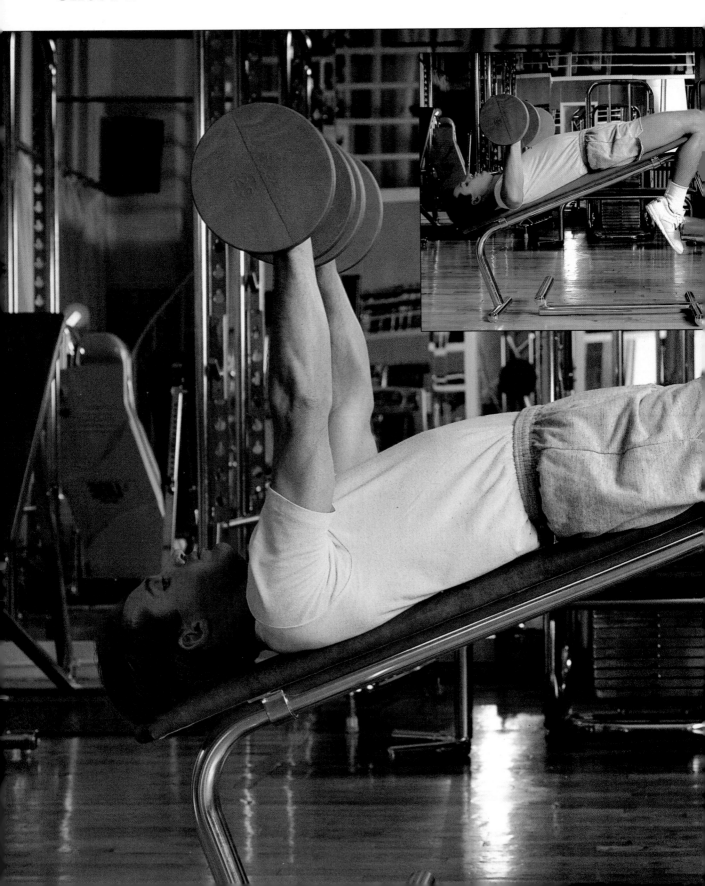

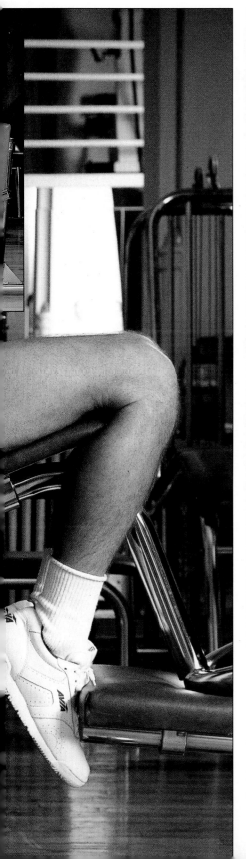

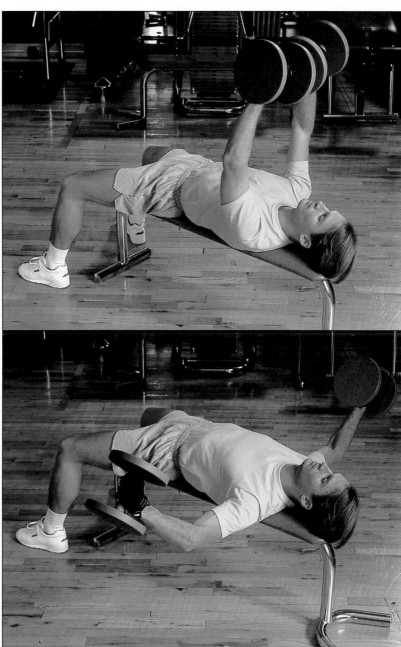

Perform a flat fly with a grip variation on a flat bench.
Lie on the bench with your feet on the floor. Extend two
dumbbells directly over your shoulders with your palms
facing away from you *(top)*. Keeping your elbows slightly
bent, slowly lower the dumbbells out to the sides *(above)*.
Return to the starting position.

To perform decline dumbbell flys, lie on a decline bench
and secure your feet. Hold two dumbbells over your
shoulders with your elbows out and your upper arms parallel
to the floor *(inset)*. Raise the dumbbells directly over your
shoulders *(left)*. Return to the starting position.

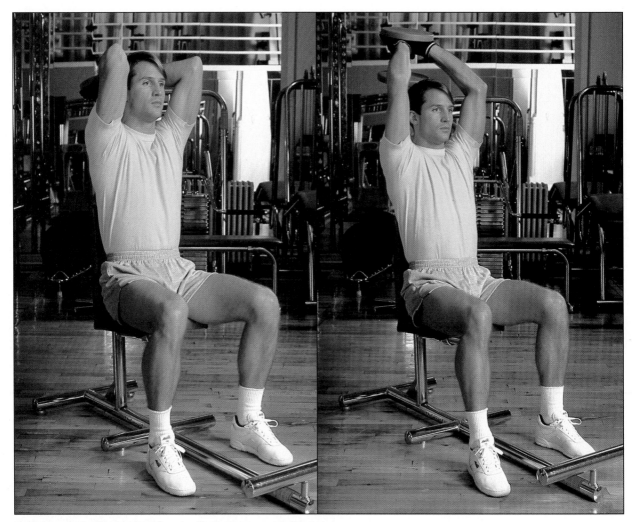

Perform seated triceps curls with a dumbbell. Sit on an exercise bench
and hold a dumbbell behind your head with both palms facing upward
(above). Keep your elbows in and lift the dumbbell over your head without locking the elbows *(above right)*. Return to the starting position.

Triceps/1

Strengthening the triceps will add muscle tone to your up-per arms and give them a harder, more well-rounded appearance. The triceps is a long muscle composed of three heads that attach to the shoulder blade and the upper arm, thus lending the muscle its name. The triceps acts to extend the elbow joint and swing the arm backward and — because it is also attached to the shoulder blade — to extend the shoulder joint. The triceps is also a stabilizing muscle; its tendons help protect both the elbow and shoulder joints from dislocation.

Since the triceps is the opposing muscle for the biceps, it should be included in any strengthening program for the biceps.

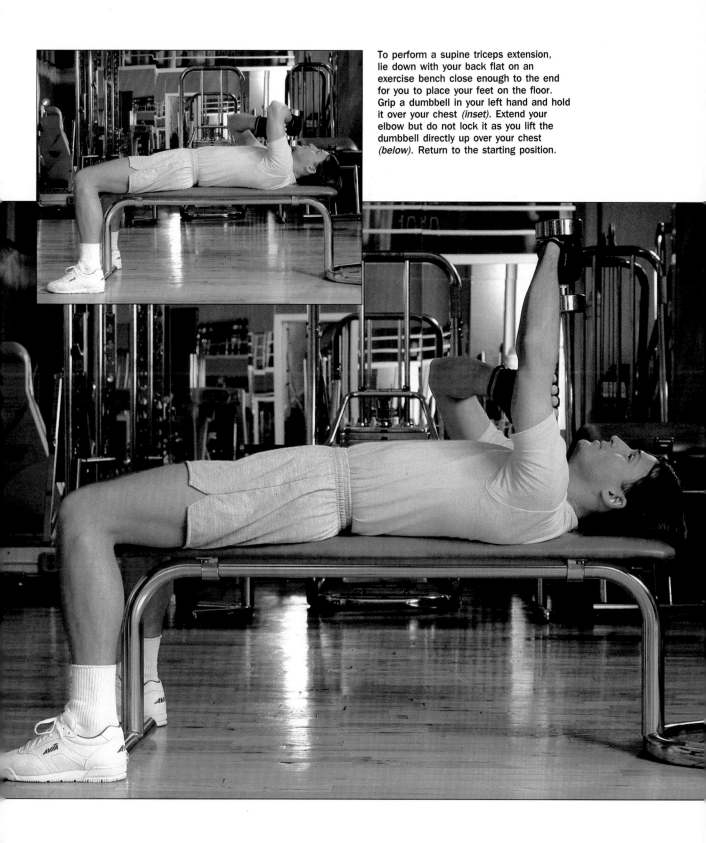

To perform a supine triceps extension, lie down with your back flat on an exercise bench close enough to the end for you to place your feet on the floor. Grip a dumbbell in your left hand and hold it over your chest *(inset)*. Extend your elbow but do not lock it as you lift the dumbbell directly up over your chest *(below)*. Return to the starting position.

Triceps/2

Perform negative triceps dips on the parallel dipping bars. Step up on a bench between the parallel bars and grip them with your elbows extended but not locked. Step off the bench and draw your feet under you *(below left)*. Keeping your elbows in, slowly release the tension and drop your body between the bars until your upper arms are parallel to the floor *(below right)*. Then step onto the bench and return to the starting position.

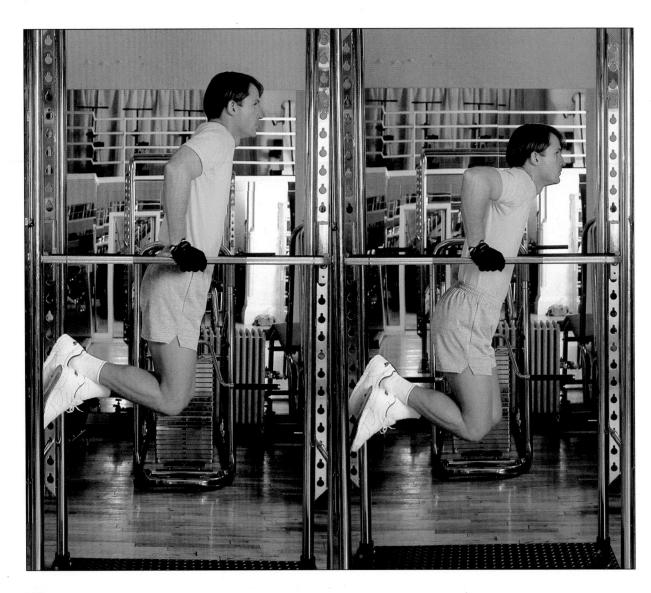

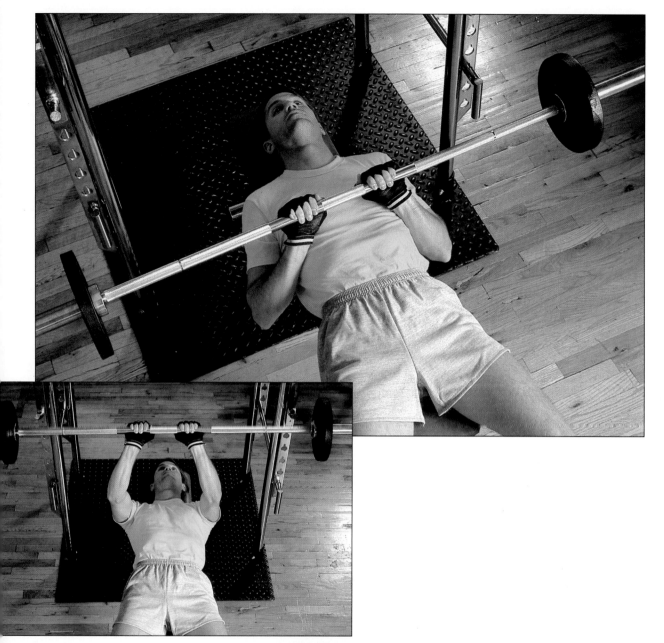

The close-grip bench press, which is similar to the triceps curl, makes an effective negative exercise. Lie supine on an exercise bench with a weighted barbell above your head on a power rack. Grasp the barbell with your palms facing up and your hands about 12 inches apart. Your partner helps you lift the barbell off the rack so that you can hold it above your shoulders with your elbows slightly bent *(inset)*. Slowly lower the barbell to within an inch of your chest *(top)*. Your partner helps you lift the barbell to the starting position.

Biceps/1

Located along the front of the upper arm, the biceps is the two-part muscle that shortens into a hard bundle when you flex your arm. Nearly everyone concerned about strength wants to condition his or her biceps, since overall muscular strength is often — though erroneously — equated with biceps strength.

The biceps bends the elbow and draws your forearm toward your upper arm. This muscle also flexes the shoulder joint so that your upper arm moves forward and turns the forearm so that your palm points upward. When the forearm's position is fixed, as when you do chin-ups, the biceps will help pull the upper arm toward the forearm.

Since the biceps turns the forearm and rotates the palm upward, you must hold the barbell, dumbbell or exercise apparatus with your palms turned upward whenever you want to exercise the biceps using the maximum work load. If your palm faces downward, other muscles will take on the work load.

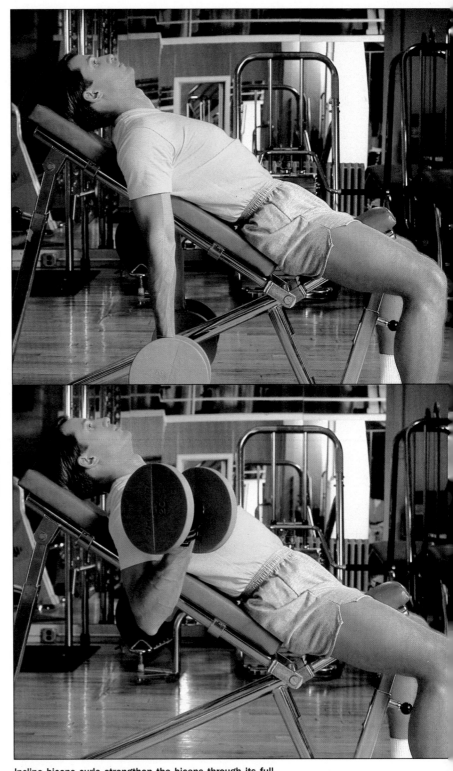

Incline biceps curls strengthen the biceps through its full range of movement. Perform them by lying on an incline board with a dumbbell in each hand and your palms facing forward. Allow each arm to hang straight down but do not lock your elbows *(top)*. Draw the dumbbells toward your shoulders *(above)*. Return to the starting position.

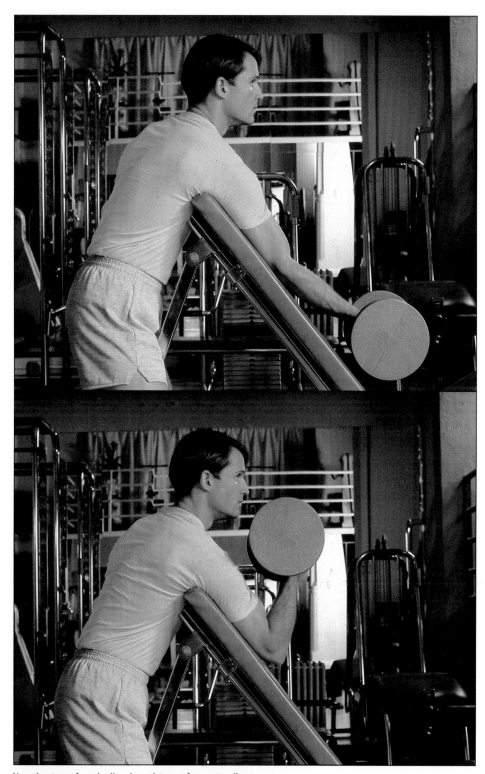

Use the top of an incline board to perform standing
preacher curls. Support your upper right arm on the incline
board with an exercise mat for a cushion. Grip a dumbbell
with your palm facing upward and your elbow slightly bent
(top). Flex your elbow and draw the dumbbell toward your
shoulder *(above)*, then return to the starting position.

Biceps/2

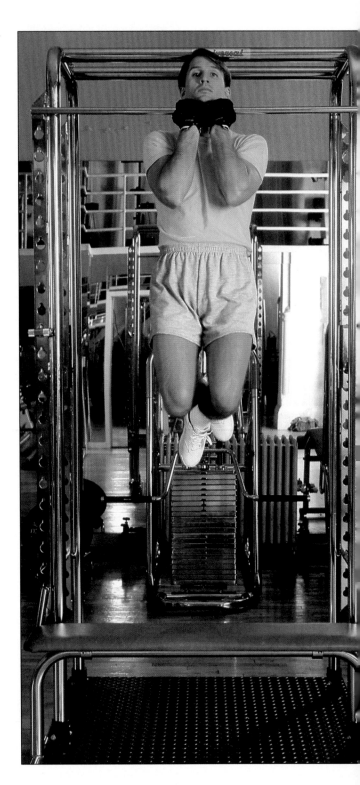

Perform close-grip negative chin-ups on a chin-up bar. Stand on a stool and grip the bar with your hands close together and your palms facing toward you. Place your chin over the bar, step off the stool and draw your legs up under you *(right)*. Slowly release the tension in your biceps so that your head drops below the level of the bar *(right center)*. Continue to release the tension slowly until your arms are extended *(far right)*. Then step back up on the stool and return to the starting position.

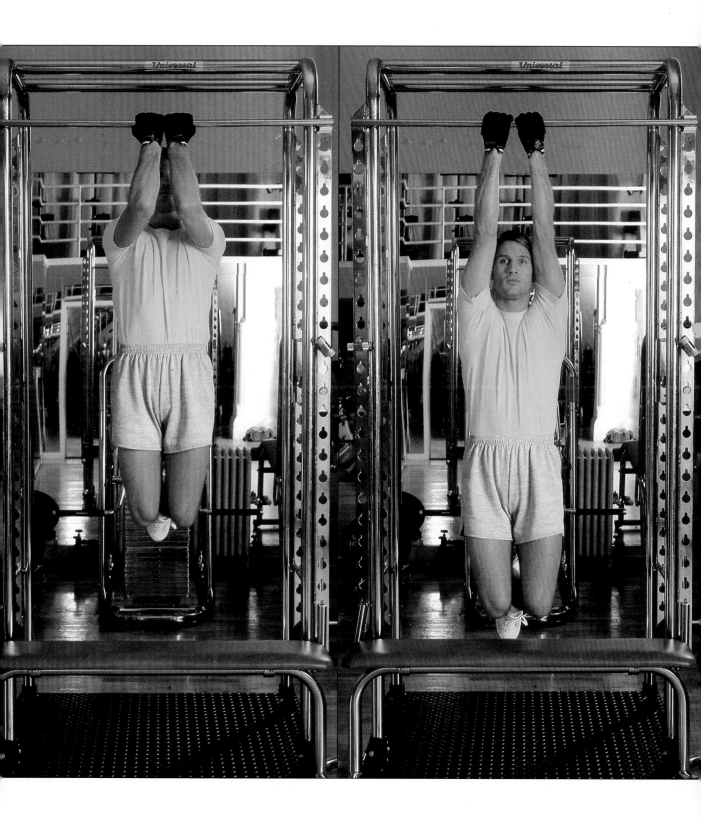

Forearms

Although building up the biceps and triceps in the upper arm is usually considered important, conditioning muscles in the lower arm is sometimes overlooked. Developing the forearm muscles not only improves the tone and shape of the arm, but also increases the power of your hand grip and the strength of your wrists.

Your wrist and hands are controlled largely by muscles in your forearms with long tendons that pass over the wrist joint. Of the approximately 20 muscles involved in wrist actions, the strongest and most important are those along the arm that extend your hand or pull it backward, and those that flex it, or draw it downward. When performing the forearm exercises, be sure to do both the flexion and the extension variations shown on this page. Both are necessary for complete forearm development.

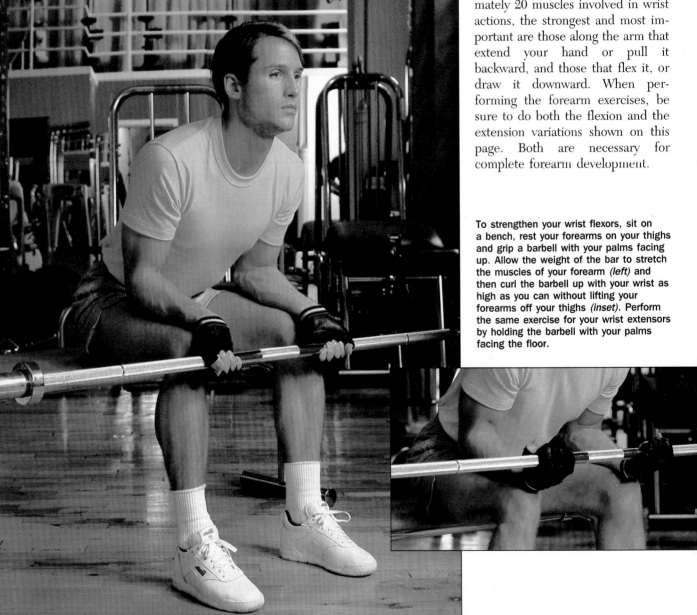

To strengthen your wrist flexors, sit on a bench, rest your forearms on your thighs and grip a barbell with your palms facing up. Allow the weight of the bar to stretch the muscles of your forearm *(left)* and then curl the barbell up with your wrist as high as you can without lifting your forearms off your thighs *(inset)*. Perform the same exercise for your wrist extensors by holding the barbell with your palms facing the floor.

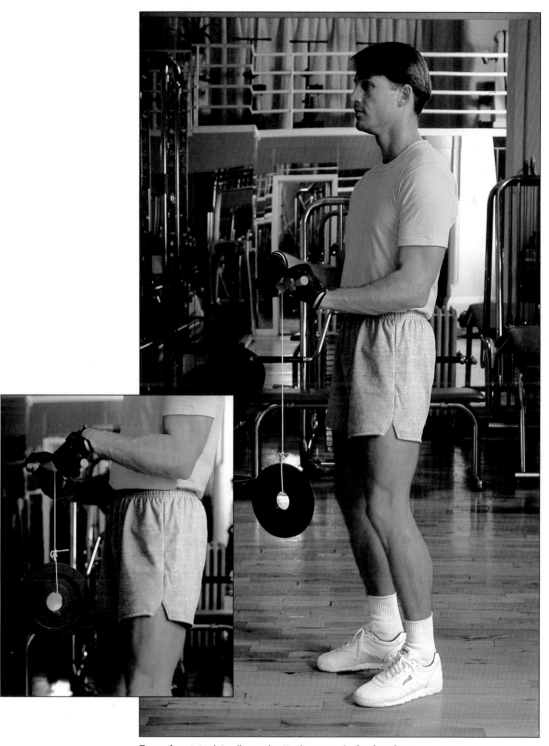

To perform a wrist roller curl, attach one end of a four-foot length of rope to a weight and the other to a section of a broom handle. Hold the handle with both palms facing down, stand erect with your knees slightly bent and keep your forearms parallel to the floor *(above)*. Turn the broom handle to roll the weight up by turning one hand at a time down over the handle *(inset)*. When the weight touches the handle, reverse the process and lower the weight to the starting position.

The open scissors crunch exercises the abdominals effectively by keeping the hip flexors and other helping muscles — which are stronger — from doing most of the work. Lie on your back with your arms at your side, palms up. Raise your right foot toward the ceiling and your left about six inches off the floor *(right)*. Lift your head and upper back off the floor and reach toward your feet, lifting your hands off the floor on the same level as your shoulders *(center right)*. Roll your back up as far as you can without straining *(bottom right)*. Return to the starting position.

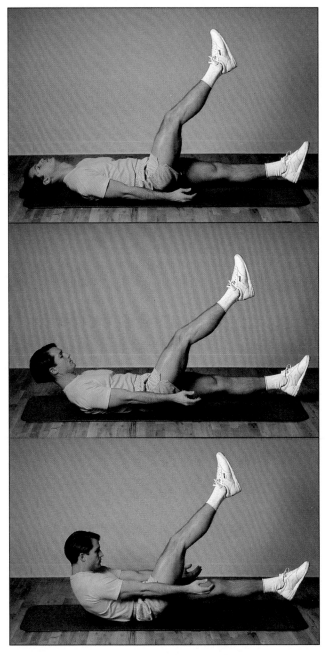

Abdominals and Lower Back/1

The small muscles of the abdominal and lower back region are sometimes neglected in weight training programs. The abdominals are especially hard to condition because they have a limited range of motion and therefore do not respond as readily as other muscles do to intense strength training.

The tendinous bands that intersect the major abdominal muscle, the rectus abdominis, lend body builders' abdomens their characteristic rippled look. This abdominal muscle originates at the bottom of the sternum and several ribs, extends along the entire length of the abdomen and attaches to the top of the pubic bone.

While the abdominals help you bend forward and draw your chest toward your pelvis, the opposing back muscles extend the back and keep it erect. The back muscles are stronger than the abdominals in most people because the back extensors are worked during many daily activities, such as standing, sitting and lifting, while the abdominals are not. When you condition your abdominal muscles in a strength training program, however, you should also strengthen the opposing back muscles so that your muscular strength is balanced.

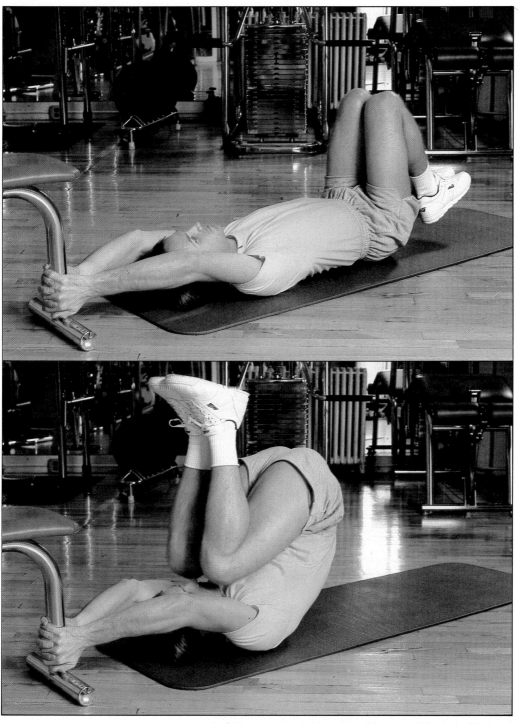

Perform a reverse sit-up to strengthen your abdominals. Lie down on your back on an exercise mat, point your knees toward the ceiling and keep your feet several inches off the floor. Reach over your head to grasp a bench or other stationary object *(top)*. Tuck your knees into your chest and roll up onto your shoulders *(bottom)*. Slowly roll back down to the starting position.

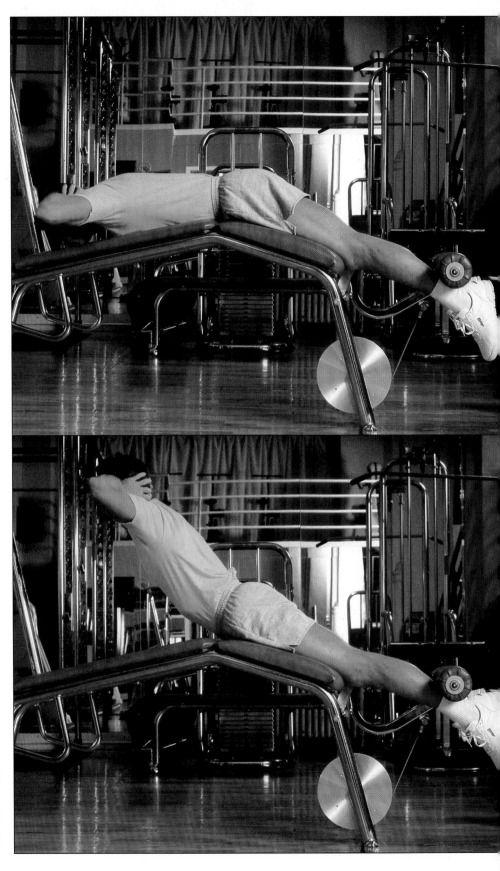

Lie face down on a leg curl machine with your ankles secured under the rollers. Interlace your fingers behind your head *(top right)*. Bring your elbows back and extend your spine as far as you can go without straining or bending your neck backward *(right)*. Slowly return to the starting position.

Abdominals and Lower Back/2

To condition your lower back and abdominals, stand erect with a barbell resting on your upper back. Stand with your head up, your chest out and your knees bent slightly *(inset)*. Keeping your head up, bend at the waist until your back is about parallel to the floor. Be sure that the barbell rests on your upper back and not on your neck *(right)*. Pause briefly and return to the starting position.

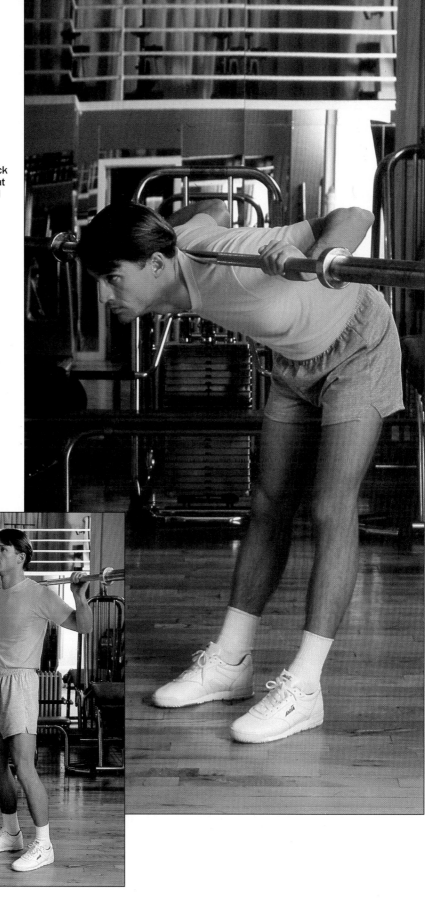

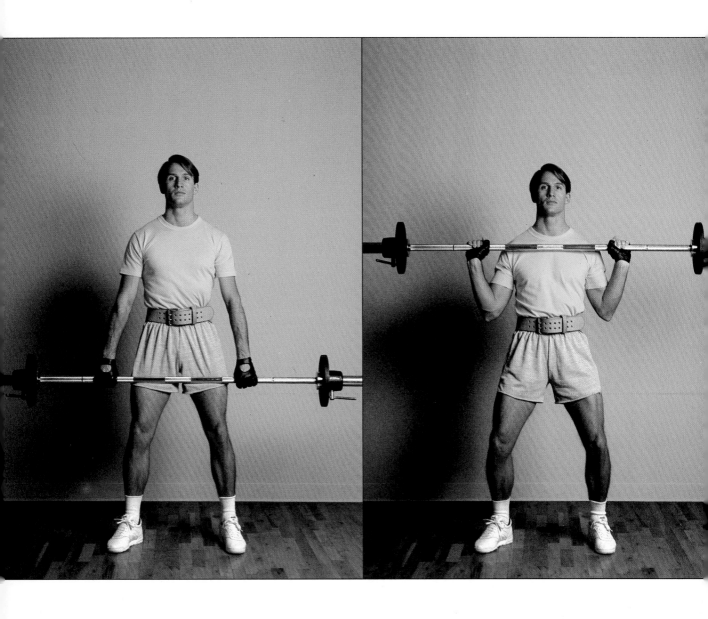

Combination Exercises/1

One of the advantages of exercising with free weights instead of machines is that you can perform one exercise to strengthen many different muscles. Two barbell exercises — the clean and press, and the push press — are particularly effective in conditioning a range of upper- and lower-body muscles. These two routines, shown here and on the following two pages, help strengthen muscles in your legs, hips, back, shoulders, triceps and biceps, as well as dozens of assisting muscles.

To perform the clean and press, stand erect while holding a barbell with your palms facing backward and your hands about two feet apart *(far left)*. Bend your elbows and use your hips to help roll the barbell up into place just above your chest *(center left)*. Do not rest the barbell on your chest but press the bar straight up, keeping your knees bent and your back straight *(above)*.

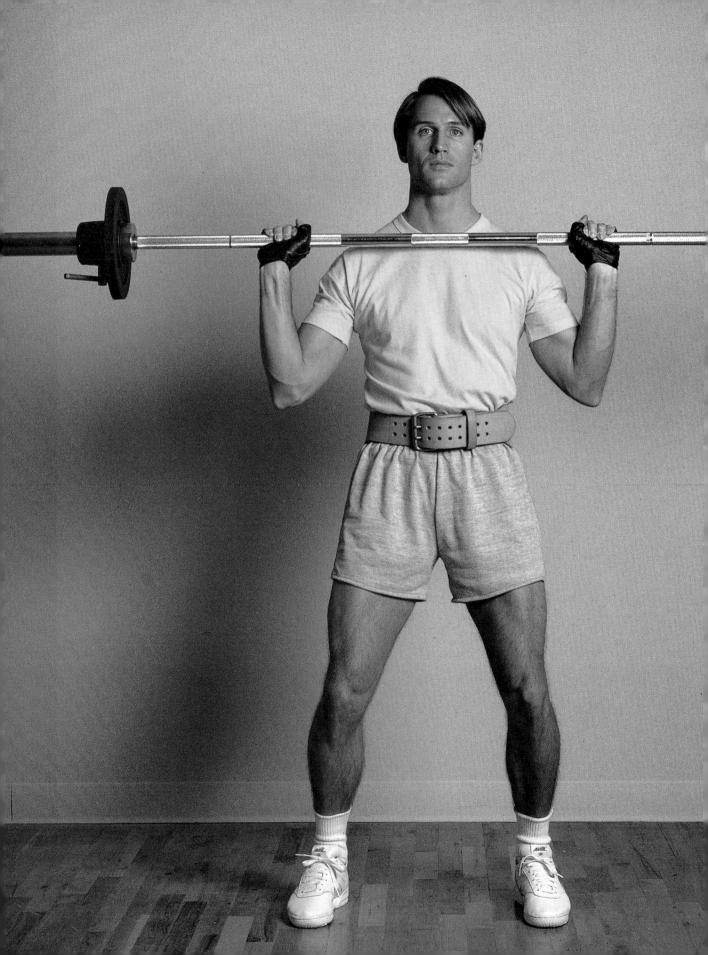

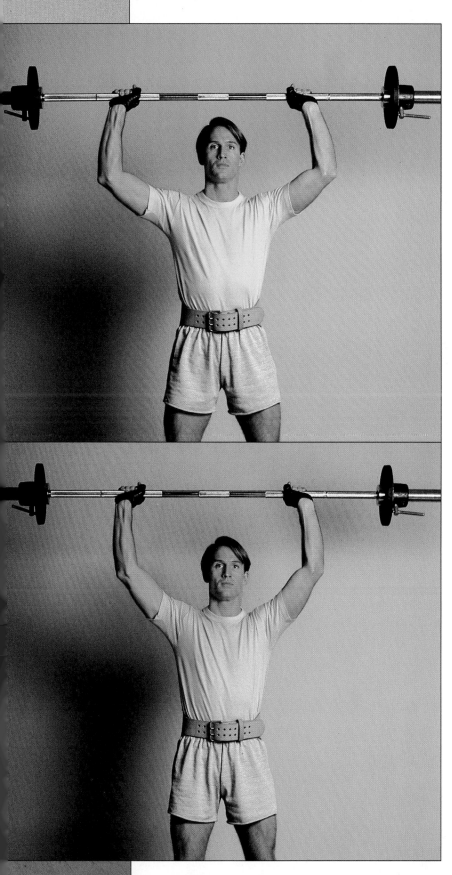

Combination
Exercises/2

Begin the push press in a half-squat
position with your knees bent, your feet
apart and the barbell on your chest
(opposite). Press the bar upward by extending your elbows. At the same time,
drive up with your legs *(top left)*. Straighten
your knees and continue to the extended
position *(bottom left)*, being sure not to
lock either your elbows or your knees.
Return to the starting position.

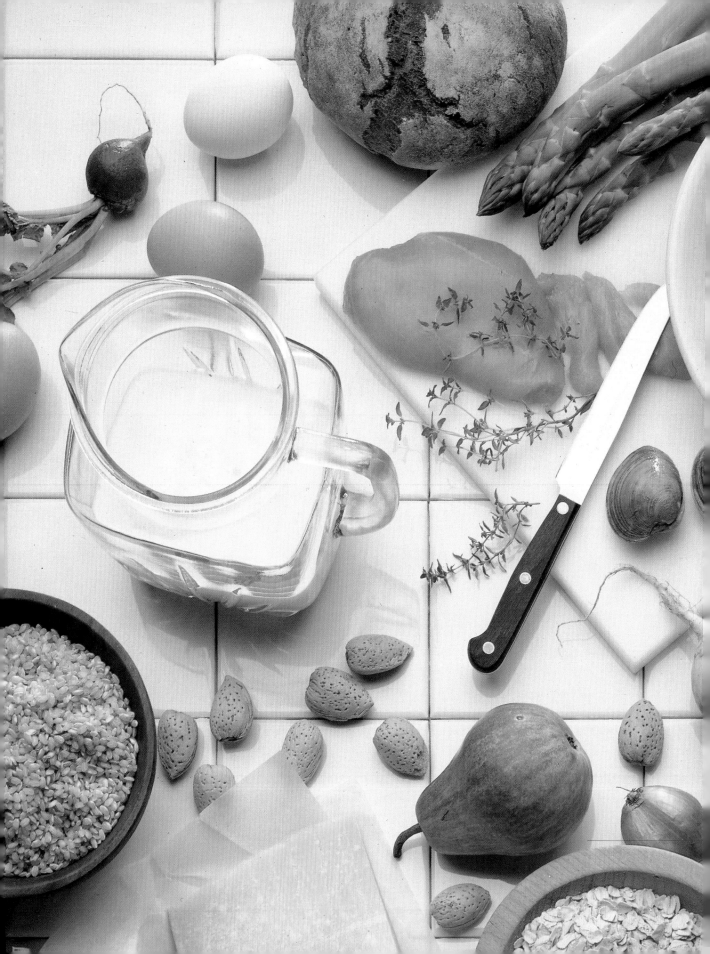

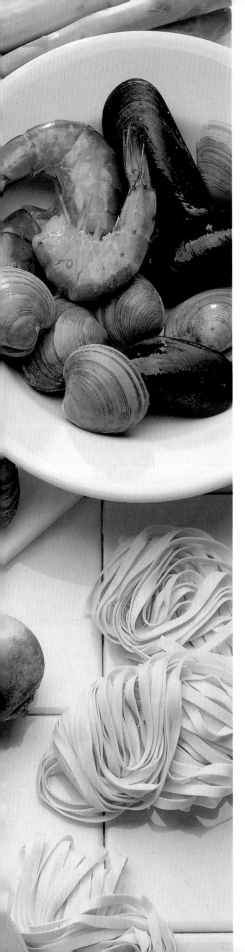

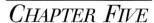
Muscle and Protein

High-quality food sources supplying all the essential amino acids

Many people, including body builders, believe that if you eat more protein, your muscles will grow larger and more powerful. In fact, muscle building occurs through complicated interactions among the foods you consume and the amount and types of exercise you perform. While muscle fibers are made mostly of protein and water, studies show that boosting protein intake without performing the kinds of muscle-building exercises demonstrated in this book will not enhance muscle growth; nor will eating extra protein increase endurance, strength or power. To build muscles, you have to combine a diet that contains adequate protein and calories with the proper exercise program. People who exercise regularly should get between 12 and 15 percent of their daily calories from protein. Consuming more than that will not contribute to greater muscle growth.

Both muscle and dietary proteins consist of 22 different chemicals called amino acids. So-called essential amino acids are the nine such chemicals that your body cannot synthesize; the other 13 amino acids can be created in your body even in the absence of dietary sources. Essential amino acids are supplied both by plant-derived foods and by foods derived from animals that eat plant foods.

The extent to which your body can use the protein in any food determines what nutritionists refer to as the quality or completeness of that protein: Foods containing all the essential acids are called high-quality or complete protein sources. With high-quality protein the essential amino acids are readily available in the right proportions to enable your body to form and repair muscles, organs, antibodies and enzymes.

As a rule, the protein in foods from animal sources is considered to be of the highest quality, since most plant-derived foods are deficient in one or more of the essential amino acids. However, plant-derived foods in certain combinations — grains with legumes, or nuts with whole grains, for example — can provide you with the complete protein that each of these foods lacks individually. Pairing plant-derived foods in this way is known as using complementary proteins. A peanut butter sandwich, in which the peanuts supply the amino acids the grains in bread lack and vice versa, is an example. Another way to enable your body to use the protein in plant-derived foods more fully is to consume them along with an animal product that contains complete protein. In the Focaccia on page 128, for example, turkey complements the protein in the whole-wheat flour.

Contrary to popular belief, red meat is not the only excellent animal source of complete protein. The best sources are those that supply the highest percentage of protein for use by the body after absorption and digestion. Poultry and fish, milk and eggs all rank as high as red meat does. To keep your fat intake low, reduce your consumption of meat and choose the leanest cuts: Although beef and pork are now raised to be less fatty than they were in the past, these meats are still high in fat and cholesterol.

The best way to keep fat to a minimum when you cook and eat poultry is to use turkey, one of the leanest meats, as well as small chickens and Cornish game hens, which are relatively low in fat; avoid duck, capon and goose, which are very fatty. White meat of poultry has less fat and cholesterol than dark meat. Before you cook poultry, remove the skin and all visible fat to cut the fat content in half.

Fish not only has less saturated fat than red meat, but it also contains oils that some scientists think can reduce the risk of heart attacks. Research indicates that substances in fish oils called omega-3 fatty acids may offer protection against heart disease. In one study performed in Holland, men who ate at least one ounce of fish every day had about one third as many fatal heart attacks as men who ate no fish. The salmon in the Smoked Salmon-Salad Sandwich on page 129 is a good source of these polyunsaturated fatty acids. While mussels, shrimp, clams and other shellfish contain fewer omega-3 fatty acids than other fish, they are relatively low in fat and calories.

The Basic Guidelines

For a moderately active adult, the National Institutes of Health recommends a diet that is low in fat, high in carbohydrates and moderate in protein. The institutes' guidelines suggest that no more than 30 percent of your calories come from fat, that 55 to 60 percent come from carbohydrates and that no more than 15 percent come from protein. A gram of fat equals nine calories, while a gram of protein or carbohydrate equals four calories; therefore, if you eat 2,100 calories a day, you should consume approximately 60 grams of fat, 315 grams of carbohydrate and no more than 75 grams of protein daily. If you follow a lowfat/high-carbohydrate diet, your chance of developing heart disease, cancer and other life-threatening diseases may be considerably reduced.

◆ The nutrition charts that accompany each of the lowfat/high-carbohydrate recipes in this book include the number of calories per serving, the number of grams of fat, carbohydrate and protein in a serving, and the percentage of calories derived from each of these nutrients. In addition, the charts provide the amount of calcium, iron and sodium per serving.

◆ Calcium deficiency may be associated with periodontal disease — which attacks the mouth's bones and tissues, including the gums — in both men and women, and with osteoporosis, or bone shrinking and weakening, in the elderly. The deficiency may also contribute to high blood pressure. The recommended daily allowance for calcium is 800 milligrams a day for men and women. Pregnant and lactating women are advised to consume 1,200 milligrams daily; a National Institutes of Health consensus panel recommends that postmenopausal women consume 1,200 to 1,500 milligrams of calcium daily.

◆ Although one way you can reduce your fat intake is to cut your consumption of red meat, you should make sure that you get your necessary iron from other sources. The Food and Nutrition Board of the National Academy of Sciences suggests a minimum of 10 milligrams of iron per day for men and 18 milligrams for women between the ages of 11 and 50.

◆ High sodium intake is associated with high blood pressure. Most adults should restrict sodium intake to between 2,000 and 2,500 milligrams a day, according to the National Academy of Sciences. One way to keep sodium consumption in check is not to add table salt to food.

Like whole milk products, skim and lowfat dairy products are the richest dietary sources of calcium, and since they too are fortified, they are high in vitamins A and D, riboflavin, thiamine, potassium, and other vitamins and minerals. The protein supplied by lowfat and skim dairy products is the same as that in whole milk products; yet skim and lowfat products are much lower in cholesterol and saturated fat. Buttermilk, lowfat yogurt and lowfat cheeses are nutritious ingredients that complement the incomplete proteins in such recipes as the Cornmeal Biscuits on page 127.

While eggs have complete protein and significant amounts of vitamin A, riboflavin, iron, phosphorus and calcium, they are high in cholesterol and saturated fat. For this reason, the American Heart Association recommends limiting consumption to two eggs per week. The recipes in this chapter provide complete, lowfat protein and relatively little cholesterol.

Breakfast

MORNING FRUIT AND YOGURT BOWL

CALORIES per serving	374
71% Carbohydrate	70 g
14% Protein	14 g
15% Fat	6 g
CALCIUM	217 mg
IRON	2 mg
SODIUM	232 mg

The combination of cottage cheese, yogurt and almonds not only provides complete protein, it also supplies one fourth of your daily calcium allowance.

1/3 cup plain lowfat yogurt
3 tablespoons lowfat cottage
  cheese (1%)
2 teaspoons brown sugar
1/2 teaspoon coconut extract
2 tablespoons rolled oats

6 almonds, coarsely chopped
1/3 cup seedless green grapes
1/3 cup strawberries
1 banana
1 tablespoon dark raisins
2 teaspoons chopped fresh mint

Process the yogurt, cottage cheese, sugar and coconut extract in a blender for about 15 seconds, or until smooth. Transfer the mixture to a bowl, cover and refrigerate. Preheat the oven to 375° F. Spread the oats and almonds on a baking sheet and toast for 5 minutes, or until golden. Remove the sheet from the oven and set aside to cool. Meanwhile, wash the grapes and strawberries, then hull and halve the strawberries. Just before serving, peel the banana and cut it into large chunks. Place the banana, grapes and strawberries in a bowl and spoon the yogurt mixture on top. Scatter the oats, almonds, raisins and mint over the yogurt and serve. Makes 1 serving

Morning Fruit and Yogurt Bowl

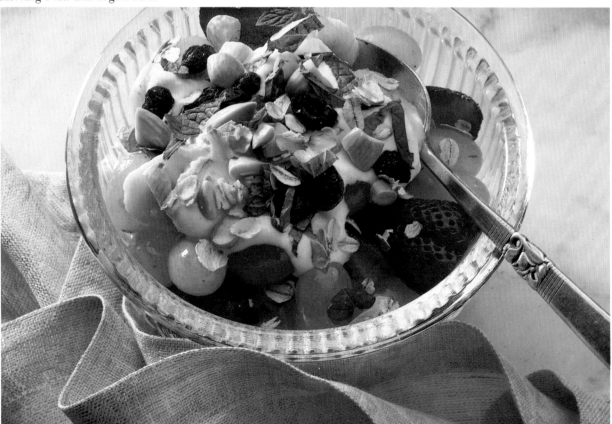

CREAMY VEGETABLE COCKTAIL

Regular cottage cheese contains at least 4 percent fat by weight; lowfat cottage cheese has the same amount of protein with one quarter the fat. The protein in cheese is of equal quality to the protein in meat.

2 medium-size red bell peppers	1/4 cup lowfat cottage cheese (1%)
1 medium-size cucumber	2 tablespoons red wine vinegar,
10 small red radishes	preferably balsamic
1/2 cup frozen corn kernels	1/4 teaspoon salt

CALORIES per serving	87
66% Carbohydrate	16 g
24% Protein	6 g
10% Fat	1 g
CALCIUM	36 mg
IRON	1 mg
SODIUM	394 mg

Preheat the broiler. To roast the bell peppers, pierce them in several places with a fork, place them on a broiler pan and broil them 6 inches from the heat for about 10 minutes, or until charred all over. Or roast the peppers directly over a burner on a gas stove, turning them until well charred all over. Place the peppers in a small paper bag, close the top and set them aside to steam for 10 minutes. Meanwhile, peel, seed and finely chop the cucumber; trim and finely chop the radishes; set aside.

Rub the charred skin off the peppers and rinse them under cold running water. Halve, seed and coarsely chop the peppers and place them in a food processor or blender with the cucumber and 1/3 cup of cold water; process for about 1 minute, or until smooth. Add the radishes, corn, cottage cheese, vinegar and salt, and process for another minute, or until smooth. Transfer the mixture to a pitcher and refrigerate it until well chilled. To serve, stir the cocktail to recombine it, then pour it into 2 tall glasses.   Makes 2 servings

CORNMEAL BISCUITS

The protein in corn lacks only two essential amino acids, lysine and tryptophane, and these are supplied in this recipe by the milk. Whole cornmeal, which retains the germ and the fiber-rich outer husk of the grain, is more nutritious than meal labeled degerminated.

2 cups unbleached all-purpose	Pinch of salt
flour, approximately	3 tablespoons butter or
2/3 cup yellow cornmeal	margarine, well chilled
1 tablespoon sugar	3/4 cup skim milk
2 teaspoons baking powder	

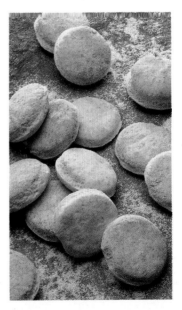

Preheat the oven to 425° F. In a medium-size bowl stir together 2 cups of flour, the cornmeal, sugar, baking powder and salt; transfer the mixture to a food processor. Cut the butter into small pieces, add it to the dry ingredients and process, pulsing the machine on and off, for about 10 seconds, or until the mixture resembles coarse meal. Add the milk and process for another 10 seconds, or until the dough forms a cohesive mass. To mix the dough by hand, cut the butter into the dry ingredients with a pastry blender or 2 knives, then add the milk and stir until combined.

Turn the dough out onto a lightly floured board and knead it gently for 30 seconds, or just until smooth. Roll it out with a floured rolling pin to a 3/4-inch thickness. Using a floured 2-inch biscuit cutter, cut out 16 biscuits and place them on a baking sheet. Reroll and cut any scraps of dough, then bake the biscuits for 10 minutes, or until golden. Serve hot.   Makes 16 biscuits

CALORIES per biscuit	104
69% Carbohydrate	18 g
10% Protein	3 g
21% Fat	2 g
CALCIUM	44 mg
IRON	1 mg
SODIUM	90 mg

Lunch

. . . .

FOCACCIA

CALORIES per serving	398
58% Carbohydrate	55 g
14% Protein	13 g
28% Fat	12 g
CALCIUM	81 mg
IRON	3 mg
SODIUM	172 mg

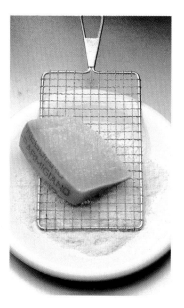

This pizza-like Italian flatbread is topped with ground turkey seasoned to taste like sausage. Cooked ground turkey has about 14 percent fat by weight, while pork sausage contains about 25 percent fat.

1 package dry yeast
3 cups unbleached all-purpose
   flour, approximately
3 tablespoons margarine, melted
   and cooled
Pinch of salt
1/4 pound ground turkey
2 garlic cloves, minced
1/4 teaspoon black pepper

1/4 teaspoon dried oregano
1 medium-size onion, sliced
1 red bell pepper
1 yellow bell pepper
2 tablespoons chopped fresh
   basil or marjoram, plus
   additional herb leaves for garnish
1 tablespoon olive oil
1/4 cup grated Parmesan

Place the yeast in a small bowl and add 1/3 cup of warm water (105-115° F); set aside for 5 minutes. Combine the yeast mixture and 1 1/2 cups of flour in a food processor and process for 5 to 10 seconds, or until a ball of dough forms. If the dough does not form a ball, with the machine running add 1 to 2 tablespoons of water and pulse the processor on and off 2 or 3 times. The dough will be tight and dry, not smooth and elastic like bread dough. Place the dough in a lightly floured bowl, cover with a damp kitchen towel and set aside in a warm place to rise for 2 hours, or until the dough is doubled in bulk.

Punch down the dough and divide it into 4 pieces. Place the dough in the food processor, add 1 1/2 cups of flour, the margarine, salt, and 1/4 cup of warm water and process for 10 to 15 seconds, or until the dough again forms a ball. If necessary, add 1 to 2 tablespoons of water as before. Return the dough to the bowl, cover and let it rise for 2 1/2 hours, or until doubled in bulk. Meanwhile, in a small bowl stir together the turkey, garlic, black pepper and oregano until well combined; cover and refrigerate.

Preheat the oven to 400° F. Peel, trim and thinly slice the onion. Stem and seed the bell peppers and cut them into slivers. Punch down the dough, form it into a ball and then flatten it into a disk. Roll it out on a lightly floured board to a 10 x 14-inch oval about 1/4 inch thick and transfer it to a baking sheet. With your fingertips make shallow indentations on the surface of the dough. Scatter the onions, bell peppers and chopped basil over the dough. Using a teaspoon, form small balls of the turkey mixture and place them on the focaccia, then sprinkle with oil and Parmesan and bake the focaccia for 15 to 20 minutes, or until the peppers begin to brown and the Parmesan is golden. Garnish with additional basil, if desired, then cut the focaccia into 6 wedges and serve.

Makes 6 servings

Note: To mix the dough by hand, combine the yeast mixture and 1 1/2 cups of flour in a large bowl. Stir until the dough forms a ball; it will be extremely tight and dry. Knead on a floured surface for 10 minutes, then return the dough to the bowl to rise. Punch down the dough, knead in the additional ingredients and knead for 5 minutes more. Return the dough to the bowl to rise.

SMOKED SALMON-SALAD SANDWICH

Fish has a higher protein-to-fat ratio than meat, and the omega-3 fatty acids in salmon may help to lower blood cholesterol.

1 cup grated carrots
1 cup grated zucchini
1/2 cup finely chopped celery
1/3 cup julienned radishes
1/4 cup finely chopped scallions
2 tablespoons finely chopped
   fresh dill
2 teaspoons Dijon-style mustard
2 teaspoons capers, rinsed
   and drained

1/2 teaspoon grated lemon peel
2 ounces thinly sliced smoked
   salmon, julienned
1/2 cup plain lowfat yogurt
2 tablespoons nonbutterfat
   sour dressing
8 sprigs watercress, trimmed of
   coarse stems
4 slices dark pumpernickel bread

In a medium-size bowl toss together the carrots, zucchini, celery, radishes, scallions and dill. Stir in the mustard, capers and lemon peel, then add the salmon, yogurt and sour dressing and stir gently to combine. Divide the watercress among the 4 slices of bread, spoon the salmon mixture on top to make open-faced sandwiches and serve immediately.   Makes 2 servings

CALORIES per serving	310
62% Carbohydrate	50 g
20% Protein	17 g
18% Fat	6 g
CALCIUM	234 mg
IRON	3 mg
SODIUM	843 mg

Focaccia

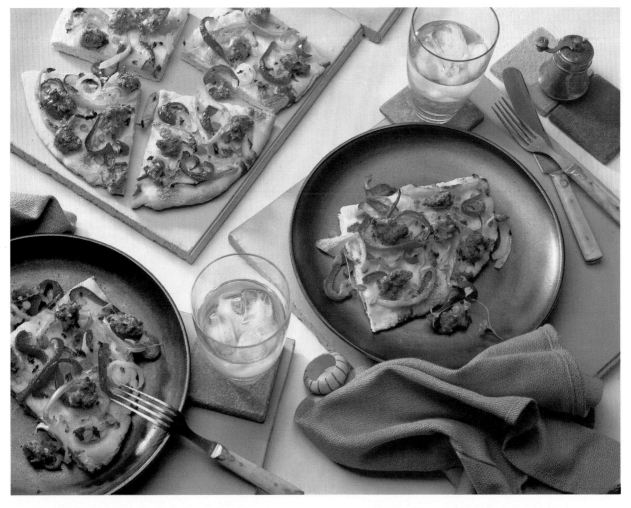

MANHATTAN CLAM CHOWDER WITH CROUTONS

This recipe shows that good amounts of iron and protein are found in foods much lower in fat than red meat. The clams, bread, potatoes and tomatoes provide most of the protein and iron in this chowder, but none of these ingredients contributes a significant amount of fat.

CALORIES per serving	179
58% Carbohydrate	27 g
17% Protein	8 g
25% Fat	5 g
CALCIUM	75 mg
IRON	6 mg
SODIUM	281 mg

2 slices whole-wheat bread
3 garlic cloves, crushed
  and peeled
24 medium-size clams in shell
3 tablespoons margarine
1 3/4 cups chopped onions
3 tablespoons unbleached
  all-purpose flour

Two 14-ounce cans plum tomatoes
3 cups unpeeled, diced
  new potatoes
1 3/4 cups diced carrots
1 bay leaf
1/4 teaspoon white pepper
1/4 cup chopped fresh parsley

Preheat the oven to 375° F. To make the croutons, rub the bread with the garlic cloves; reserve the garlic. Cut the bread into 1/2-inch cubes, spread them on a baking sheet and bake for 5 to 10 minutes, or until golden. Remove the croutons from the oven and set aside.

Thoroughly scrub the clams and rinse them in several changes of cold water. Bring 2 cups of water to a boil in a large saucepan over medium-high heat. Add the clams, cover the pot and cook for 3 minutes. Uncover the pot, stir the clams and remove any whose shells have opened, placing them in a large bowl. Cover the pan and continue cooking the remaining clams for 7 minutes, opening the pan frequently to stir them and removing any opened clams each time. After the clams have cooked for 10 minutes, transfer the remaining opened clams to a large bowl and remove and discard any unopened clams. Cover the bowl loosely with foil and set aside. Strain the cooking liquid through a fine strainer and set aside; you should have about 2 cups of clam stock. Rinse and dry the pan.

Melt the margarine in the saucepan over medium heat. Add the onions, and cook, stirring, for 3 to 5 minutes, or until softened. Stir in the flour, and cook for 1 minute, or until the flour is incorporated. Gradually stir in the tomatoes and their liquid, bring the mixture to a boil and cook, stirring constantly, for 2 to 3 minutes, or until thickened. Add the potatoes, carrots, bay leaf, garlic cloves, clam stock and 1 cup of water. Cover the pan, reduce the heat to low and simmer the chowder, stirring occasionally, for 20 to 25 minutes. Meanwhile, shuck the clams and discard the shells. Add any clam juice remaining in the bowl to the chowder. Coarsely chop the clams; set aside.

Just before serving, add the pepper to the chowder and remove and discard the bay leaf. Divide the clams among 8 bowls and ladle the chowder over them. Top each serving of chowder with croutons and sprinkle with parsley.

Makes 8 servings

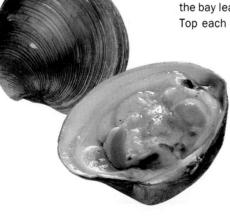

CHICKEN CLUB SANDWICH WITH CARROT SALAD

This sandwich provides about half the protein needed daily by a 130-pound adult. It also provides half the daily allowance of vitamin C.

CALORIES per serving	426
63% Carbohydrate	69 g
20% Protein	24 g
17% Fat	9 g
CALCIUM	160 mg
IRON	5 mg
SODIUM	867 mg

1 1/2 tablespoons reduced-calorie mayonnaise
1 1/2 tablespoons plain lowfat yogurt
1 1/2 cups shredded carrots
1/3 cup golden raisins
1 teaspoon lemon juice
1/2 teaspoon grated lemon peel
1 tablespoon spicy brown mustard
2 thin slices Canadian bacon
4 leaves Romaine lettuce
1 medium-size tomato, sliced
1/2 medium-size onion, sliced
2 ounces skinless cooked chicken breast, thinly sliced
6 slices whole-wheat bread

Mix the mayonnaise and yogurt in a cup. For the carrot salad, in a small bowl stir together the carrots, raisins, lemon juice, lemon peel and half the mayonnaise mixture. Cover the bowl and refrigerate until ready to serve. Stir the mustard into the remaining mayonnaise mixture, cover and refrigerate.

Cook the bacon in a small nonstick skillet over medium heat for 1 minute on each side, or until heated through; set aside. Divide the Romaine, tomato and onion into 4 portions and the chicken and bacon into 2 portions.

Toast the bread and spread one side of each slice with the mayonnaise mixture. To assemble each sandwich, top 1 slice of toast with 1 portion of Romaine, tomato, onion and chicken; place another slice of toast on top. Add another portion of Romaine, tomato and onion, and top with bacon and the last slice of toast. Insert 2 long toothpicks or thin wooden skewers into each sandwich. Using a sharp serrated knife, cut the sandwiches diagonally in half. Serve the sandwiches with the carrot salad. Makes 2 servings

RICE VICHYSSOISE

The protein in this soup is about evenly divided between animal and vegetable sources. When the two are balanced in this way, the protein in the plant foods is more fully utilized by the body.

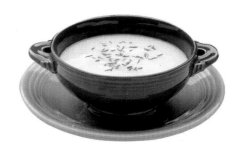

1 tablespoon plus 1 teaspoon butter or margarine
3 cups chopped leeks, white part only
3 cups low-sodium chicken stock
1 cup white rice
1/4 teaspoon white pepper
1 cup skim milk
1 tablespoon chopped chives

CALORIES per serving	303
73% Carbohydrate	54 g
11% Protein	8 g
16% Fat	6 g
CALCIUM	135 mg
IRON	4 mg
SODIUM	129 mg

Heat the butter in a medium-size saucepan over medium heat. Add the leeks and sauté for 2 to 3 minutes, or until softened. Add the stock, rice, pepper and 3 1/2 cups of water and bring to a boil over medium heat. Cover the pan, reduce the heat to low and simmer the soup for 30 minutes.

Remove the pan from the heat and let the soup cool slightly, then process it in a food processor or blender for about 30 seconds, or until smooth. With the machine running, gradually add the milk. Reheat the soup briefly over low heat, then divide it among 4 bowls, sprinkle it with chives and serve. Or refrigerate the soup until well chilled and serve it cold. Makes 4 servings

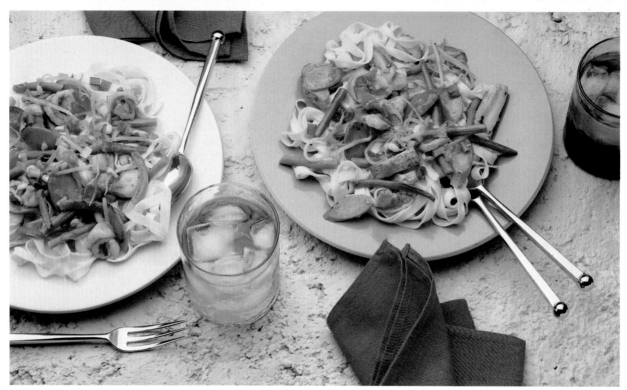

Stir-Fried Vegetables and
Shrimp on Fettuccine

Dinner
. . . .

STIR-FRIED VEGETABLES AND SHRIMP ON FETTUCCINE

This pasta and seafood dish is a good source of protein. It also supplies iron and potassium as well as vitamins A, B complex and C.

1/2 pound green beans	1/2 pound fettuccine
1/2 pound yellow squash	1/4 pound bean sprouts
1/4 pound carrots	1/2 cup low-sodium chicken stock
6 ounces shelled, deveined shrimp (about 14 medium-size shrimp)	2 teaspoons tamari
2 tablespoons vegetable oil	2 teaspoons cornstarch
2 teaspoons minced garlic	2/3 cup chopped scallions
4 thin slices fresh ginger	1 tablespoon plus 1 teaspoon margarine

Wash and trim the beans, squash and carrots. Cut the beans into 2-inch lengths, the squash into 2-inch sticks 1/4 inch thick and the carrots into 1/4-inch-thick diagonal slices. Slice the shrimp in half lengthwise; set aside.

Heat 1 tablespoon of oil in a medium-size skillet over medium heat until very hot but not smoking. Add the shrimp, 1 teaspoon of garlic and 2 slices of ginger and stir-fry for about 2 minutes, or until the shrimp turn orange. Transfer the shrimp, garlic and ginger to a bowl; cover loosely and set aside. Wipe out the skillet with paper towels.

Bring 3 quarts of water to a boil in a large pot over medium-high heat. Cook

CALORIES per serving	416
55% Carbohydrate	57 g
19% Protein	20 g
26% Fat	13 g
CALCIUM	97 mg
IRON	4 mg
SODIUM	257 mg

the fettuccine for 10 to 12 minutes, or according to the package directions, until al dente Meanwhile, heat the remaining oil in the skillet over medium-high heat. Add the remaining garlic and ginger, the beans, squash, carrots and bean sprouts, and cook, stirring, for 2 minutes, or until the vegetables are crisp-tender. Mix the stock, tamari and cornstarch in a cup, add the mixture to the vegetables and bring to a boil, stirring constantly. Add the shrimp and scallions, and stir to combine. Remove the pan from the heat and set aside.

Drain the fettuccine thoroughly, return it to the pot and toss it with the margarine until well coated. Divide the fettuccine among 4 plates and top it with the shrimp and vegetables. Makes 4 servings

Note: Tamari, a mellow, unrefined soy sauce, is sold in health-food stores.

SHERRIED CHICKEN AND RICE

Removing the skin from poultry eliminates half the fat but does not affect the protein content of the meat. Chicken is an excellent source of niacin, a B vitamin that helps the body metabolize protein.

CALORIES per serving	263
55% Carbohydrate	37 g
18% Protein	13 g
27% Fat	7 g
CALCIUM	62 mg
IRON	2 mg
SODIUM	141 mg

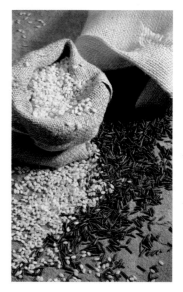

2 tablespoons wild rice

1 cup brown rice

1 tablespoon cornstarch

1/4 teaspoon coarsely ground black pepper

Pinch of salt

1/2 pound skinless, boneless chicken breast

3 tablespoons margarine

5 shallots, minced

3 garlic cloves, minced

1 tablespoon dry sherry

1 tablespoon chopped fresh thyme, or 1 teaspoon dried thyme

2 cups thinly sliced cabbage

2 cups thinly sliced carrots

2 cups thinly sliced zucchini

2 tablespoons chopped fresh dill

Rinse the wild rice in a small strainer under cold running water. In a medium-size saucepan combine the wild rice, brown rice and 2 cups of water and bring to a boil over medium-high heat. Cover the pan, reduce the heat to low and simmer for 40 minutes, or until the rice is tender and the water is completely absorbed. Meanwhile, combine the cornstarch, pepper and salt on a sheet of waxed paper; set aside. Trim and discard any fat from the chicken and cut the chicken into 2 x 1/2-inch strips. Gently toss the chicken strips in the cornstarch mixture until coated; set aside.

Melt 1 1/2 tablespoons of margarine in a medium-size nonstick skillet over medium-high heat. Add the shallots and half the garlic and sauté for 15 seconds. Add the chicken and cook for 30 seconds without stirring, then cook, stirring constantly, for another 2 to 3 minutes. Add the sherry, half the thyme and 1/2 cup of water, cover the pan, reduce the heat to medium-low and cook for 1 minute. Transfer the chicken to a bowl, cover loosely with plastic wrap and set aside. Rinse and dry the skillet.

Melt the remaining margarine in the skillet over medium-high heat. Add the remaining garlic and thyme, the cabbage, carrots and zucchini, and cook, stirring constantly, for 2 to 3 minutes. Add 1/4 cup of water, cover the pan and cook for another minute, or until the cabbage is wilted and the carrots are tender. Return the chicken to the skillet and cook, stirring, for 1 minute more.

To serve, stir the dill into the rice. Divide the rice among 6 plates and spoon the chicken mixture on top. Makes 6 servings

MUSHROOM-VEGETABLE BARLEY

CALORIES per serving	344
64% Carbohydrate	56 g
10% Protein	9 g
26% Fat	10 g
CALCIUM	76 mg
IRON	4 mg
SODIUM	134 mg

Barley is a good source of B vitamins and of minerals, including potassium and phosphorus. It is nearly 10 percent protein, and the amino acid it lacks is supplied in this dish by the chicken stock and cheese.

1 cup barley
1 cup low-sodium chicken stock
1 ounce dried shiitake or
  porcini mushrooms
3 tablespoons butter
1/4 pound fresh mushrooms,
  washed and trimmed

2 cups thinly sliced snow peas
1 1/2 cups thinly sliced red or
  yellow bell peppers
3/4 cup chopped onion
1/4 cup chopped fresh parsley
1/4 teaspoon black pepper
1 tablespoon grated Parmesan

Rinse the barley in a strainer under cold running water. Place the barley, stock and 2 cups of water in a medium-size saucepan, and bring to a boil over medium heat. Cover the pan, reduce the heat to medium-low and cook for 45 minutes. Meanwhile, place the dried mushrooms in a small bowl, add 1 cup of hot water and set aside to soak.

When the barley has cooked for 45 minutes, strain the mushroom-soaking liquid and add the dried mushrooms and liquid to the pan. Cook the barley for 15 minutes more. Meanwhile, melt the butter in a medium-size skillet over medium heat. Add the fresh mushrooms, snow peas, bell peppers and onion, and cook, stirring constantly, for 5 minutes. Add the barley, parsley and black pepper and stir to combine. Sprinkle the Parmesan over the barley and vegetables and divide the mixture among 4 plates.   Makes 4 servings

ORIENTAL MUSSEL STEW

CALORIES per serving	321
74% Carbohydrate	60 g
15% Protein	12 g
11% Fat	4 g
CALCIUM	72 mg
IRON	4 mg
SODIUM	200 mg

In addition to providing 4 milligrams of iron, this stew is a good source of vitamin C, which helps the body absorb the iron. Most of the vitamin C comes from the orange juice; the rest is in the watercress, snow peas and onions.

1/2 ounce dried shiitake
  mushrooms
6 ounces snow peas
2 medium-size onions
1 cup packed watercress sprigs
1 cup orange juice
1 cup white wine
2 teaspoons reduced-sodium
  soy sauce
2 teaspoons Oriental sesame oil
1 low-sodium chicken
  bouillon cube

1 tablespoon julienned
  fresh ginger
1/2 teaspoon anise seed
12 medium-size mussels in shell
  (14 ounces), scrubbed and
  debearded
5 ounces fresh vermicelli
3/4 cup drained, sliced
  water chestnuts
1 cup drained canned baby corn
2 tablespoons chopped fresh
  coriander

Place the mushrooms in a small bowl, add 3/4 cup of hot water and set aside to soak for 30 minutes. Meanwhile, trim the snow peas and cut them in half diagonally. Peel, trim and very thinly sliver the onions. Trim and discard the tough stems from the watercress; set aside.

Reserving the liquid, trim and discard the stems from the mushrooms and cut the caps into julienne strips. In a large saucepan combine the mushrooms, orange juice, wine, soy sauce, sesame oil, bouillon cube, ginger, anise seed and 1 quart of water. Strain and add the mushroom-soaking liquid, bring the mixture to a boil over medium heat and simmer for 15 minutes. Meanwhile, divide the watercress among 4 soup bowls; set aside. Add the mussels to the pan and cook for 1 minute, then add the onions, vermicelli and water chestnuts, and cook for another 2 minutes. Add the snow peas and corn and cook for another minute, or until the vermicelli is tender. Remove the pan from the heat and stir in the coriander, then ladle the soup over the watercress and serve immediately.   Makes 4 servings

Note: If fresh vermicelli is unavailable, use dried vermicelli or spaghettini, broken into short lengths and precooked for 5 minutes.

STUFFED SQUASH WITH CHEESE

Acorn squash is an excellent source of potassium. An important mineral for anyone who works out regularly, potassium helps regulate the contractions of the muscles, including the heart.

CALORIES per serving	364
58% Carbohydrate	56 g
11% Protein	10 g
31% Fat	13 g
CALCIUM	259 mg
IRON	3 mg
SODIUM	234 mg

2 medium-size acorn squash
  (about 3 pounds total weight)
3 tablespoons butter or margarine
1 tablespoon minced garlic
1 cup peeled, diced eggplant
1 cup diced red bell pepper
2 cups cooked brown rice
  (2/3 cup raw)

1/4 cup chopped fresh parsley
1 tablespoon balsamic vinegar
3/4 teaspoon dried
  oregano, crumbled
1/4 teaspoon pepper
Pinch of salt
3/4 cup grated part skim-milk
  mozzarella

Preheat the oven to 375° F. Using a large, heavy knife, carefully halve the squash lengthwise. Place the halves cut side down on a foil-lined baking sheet and bake for 20 minutes, or until the flesh is barely tender. (The squash will be cooked further after it is stuffed.) Leave the oven at 375° F.

Let the squash cool slightly, then remove and discard the seeds and stringy membranes. Using a teaspoon, scoop out and reserve the flesh, leaving a 1/4-inch-thick shell and being careful not to pierce the skin; set aside the flesh and hollowed-out squash.

For the stuffing, melt 2 tablespoons of butter in a medium-size skillet over medium heat. Add the garlic and sauté for 15 seconds, then add the eggplant and sauté for 2 to 3 minutes, or until the eggplant begins to soften. Add the bell pepper and continue cooking, stirring occasionally, for 2 minutes. Add the remaining butter, the reserved squash flesh, the rice, parsley, vinegar, oregano, pepper and salt, and stir to combine thoroughly. Divide the mixture among the squash shells, top with mozzarella and bake for 10 to 15 minutes, or until the filling is heated through.   Makes 4 servings

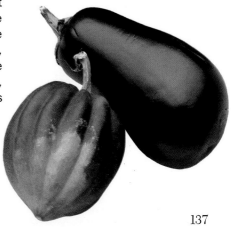

Dessert

PHYLLO FIG PASTRIES

Almonds, like most nuts, have a high percentage of protein, and they contain more calcium than any other type of nuts.

CALORIES per pastry	113
70% Carbohydrate	20 g
8% Protein	2 g
22% Fat	3 g
CALCIUM	23 mg
IRON	1 mg
SODIUM	27 mg

1/2 ounce chopped almonds
   (about 12 whole almonds)
1 almond herbal tea bag
1 Granny Smith apple
3 ounces dried figs

1/2 teaspoon almond extract
4 zwieback biscuits, crumbled
4 sheets phyllo
1 tablespoon margarine, melted
   and cooled

Preheat the oven to 375° F. Spread the almonds on a baking sheet and toast them for 5 minutes, or until golden. Meanwhile, bring 1/2 cup of water to a boil in a small nonreactive saucepan. Place the tea bag in the saucepan and set aside to steep. Core and grate the unpeeled apple. Remove the almonds from the oven and set them aside to cool. Leave the oven at 375° F.

Discard the tea bag, then add the figs and almond extract to the pan and bring to a boil over medium-high heat. Reduce the heat to low, cover and cook for 25 minutes, or until the figs are tender and most of the liquid is absorbed. Using a slotted spoon, transfer the figs to a food processor and process until coarsely chopped. Add the apple and zwieback and process just until combined, then stir in the almonds. (To make the filling by hand, mash the figs, chop them with the apple and zwieback, then stir in the almonds.)

Phyllo Fig Pastries

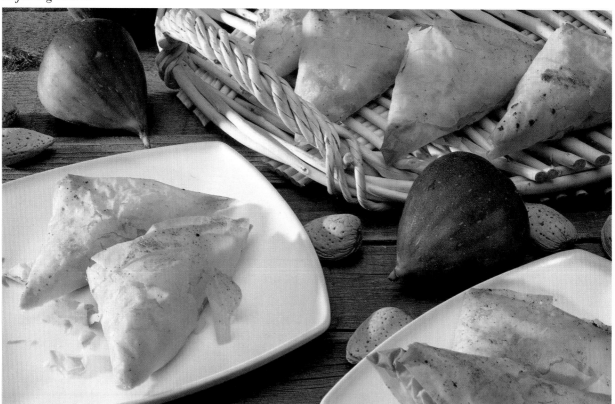

Cut each phyllo sheet in half to form two 8 x 12-inch sheets. Place a sheet on the work surface and fold it in half to form a 4 x 12-inch strip with a narrow end toward you. (Cover the remaining sheets with a damp kitchen towel so they do not dry out.) Place 1/4 cup of filling at the bottom of the folded strip, then fold up a corner of the phyllo diagonally to form a triangle. Continue folding it diagonally to the top of the strip to form a triangular packet. Place the packet on a foil-lined baking sheet and cover it loosely with plastic wrap. Make 7 more packets in the same fashion. Remove the plastic wrap, brush the pastries with margarine and bake for 12 minutes, or until golden. Transfer the pastries to a rack to cool for 5 minutes before serving.   Makes 8 pastries

BLUEBERRY-BUTTERMILK FREEZE

A cup of strawberry ice cream has approximately the same amount of protein as this berry freeze, but the ice cream may contain three times as much fat.

1 cup fresh or frozen blueberries	1 teaspoon vanilla extract
1/4 cup sugar	1 2/3 cups buttermilk
2 tablespoons chopped fresh mint	1/4 cup lowfat sour cream

Purée the blueberries in a food processor or blender. Add the sugar, mint and vanilla and process for another 5 seconds. With the machine running, add the buttermilk and sour cream and process for 30 seconds more. Turn the mixture into a shallow pan and place it in the freezer for 2 hours, or until slushy.

Return the mixture to the food processor or blender, in 2 batches if necessary, and process it for 10 seconds to break up the ice, then return it to the pan and freeze it for 4 hours more, or until firm. If necessary, let the blueberry freeze soften at room temperature for 15 minutes before serving.

Makes 4 servings

CALORIES per serving	133
73% Carbohydrate	25 g
14% Protein	5 g
13% Fat	2 g
CALCIUM	142 mg
IRON	.2 mg
SODIUM	130 mg

FRUIT WITH SHERRY CUSTARD SAUCE

This dessert supplies 10 milligrams of protein. The complete protein in the eggs and milk lets you get the full benefit of the protein in the nuts and fruit.

2 tablespoons pine nuts	2 egg yolks
4 cups fresh blueberries	1/2 cup sugar
4 cups hulled, halved strawberries	1 cup evaporated skimmed milk
1/2 cup slivered dried apricots	1 1/2 tablespoons dry sherry

Heat a small skillet over medium heat. Place the pine nuts in the skillet and toast them, shaking the pan, for about 2 minutes, or until the nuts are golden; remove the skillet from the heat and set aside.

In a large bowl gently toss together the blueberries, strawberries and apricots; set aside. For the custard, in a small saucepan whisk together the egg yolks and sugar, then stir in the milk. Heat the mixture over medium heat, stirring constantly, for about 8 minutes, or until thickened. Stir in the sherry and cook for 1 minute more; remove the pan from the heat and set aside.

To serve, divide the fruit mixture among 4 dessert dishes. Spoon the custard over the fruit and sprinkle with pine nuts.   Makes 4 servings

CALORIES per serving	369
76% Carbohydrate	75 g
10% Protein	10 g
14% Fat	6 g
CALCIUM	237 mg
IRON	3 mg
SODIUM	90 mg

Snacks

APPLE CINNAMON CUPCAKES

CALORIES per cupcake	193
62% Carbohydrate	30 g
8% Protein	4 g
30% Fat	6 g
CALCIUM	72 mg
IRON	1 mg
SODIUM	176 mg

Cupcakes can be more than empty calories when they are made with nutritious ingredients like oats, apples, buttermilk and yogurt.

1 cup unbleached all-purpose flour
1 teaspoon baking powder
3/4 teaspoon ground cinnamon
1/2 teaspoon baking soda
Pinch of salt
1 cup rolled oats
1/2 cup buttermilk

1/2 cup plain lowfat yogurt
2 eggs, beaten
1 cup chopped dried apples
  (2 ounces)
2/3 cup packed brown sugar
5 tablespoons butter, melted
  and cooled

Preheat the oven to 375° F. Line 12 standard-size or 24 miniature muffin tin cups with paper liners; set aside. In a small bowl combine the flour, baking powder, cinnamon, baking soda and salt. In a medium-size bowl stir together the oats, buttermilk and yogurt. In a large bowl stir together the eggs, apples, sugar and butter, then add the buttermilk mixture and stir to combine. Fold in the dry ingredients just until incorporated and divide the batter among the muffin tin cups. Bake for 20 minutes (12 to 14 minutes for miniature cupcakes), or until a toothpick inserted in the center of a cupcake comes out clean and the tops are golden brown.   Makes 12 standard-size cupcakes

OATMEAL SCONES

CALORIES per scone	198
62% Carbohydrate	30 g
8% Protein	5 g
30% Fat	7 g
CALCIUM	37 mg
IRON	1 mg
SODIUM	201 mg

Scones are usually made with cream, but in this recipe lowfat buttermilk is used instead. The milk also provides the amino acid missing in the oats.

1 1/3 cups unbleached all-purpose
  flour, approximately
1 cup rolled oats
1 tablespoon sugar
1 teaspoon baking soda

Pinch of salt
1/4 cup butter, well chilled
2/3 cup buttermilk
1/3 cup golden raisins

Preheat the oven to 400° F. In a food processor combine 1 1/3 cups of flour, the oats, sugar, baking soda and salt. Cut the butter into small pieces, add it to the dry ingredients and process, pulsing the machine on and off, for 10 seconds, or until the mixture resembles coarse meal. Add the buttermilk and process for another 10 seconds, or until the dough forms a ball. To mix by hand, cut the butter into the dry ingredients with a pastry blender or 2 knives, then add the buttermilk and stir until the dough forms a ball.

  Turn the dough out onto a lightly floured board and gently knead in the raisins for 1 minute, or until the dough is smooth. Using a lightly floured rolling pin, roll the dough out into an 8 1/2-inch disk about 1/2 inch thick. Place it on a baking sheet and with a sharp knife lightly score it into 8 wedges. (For scones with an all-over crust, cut the wedges apart completely and place them 1 inch apart.) Bake for 15 minutes, or until golden. Cool slightly, then cut the scones along the scored lines.   Makes 8 scones

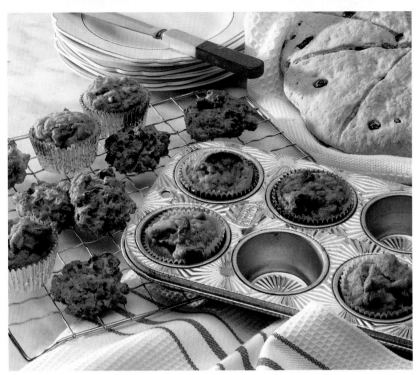

Apple Cinnamon Cupcakes, Butternut Squash Hermits, Oatmeal Scones

BUTTERNUT SQUASH HERMITS

Comparable cookie recipes may have four times as much shortening and six times as much sugar as this one.

1 cup cooked butternut squash,
   or 3/4 pound uncooked
   butternut squash
Vegetable cooking spray
1 cup unbleached all-purpose flour
1 cup rolled oats
1 teaspoon baking soda
3/4 teaspoon ground ginger

1/4 teaspoon ground allspice
Pinch of salt
1/4 cup margarine, softened
1/3 cup brown sugar
1 egg
1/2 teaspoon vanilla extract
1/2 cup each diced dried apricots,
   dried currants and prunes

If using uncooked squash, preheat the oven to 375° F. Using a large, heavy knife, carefully halve the squash lengthwise. Place the halves cut side down on a foil-lined baking sheet and bake for 25 minutes, or until tender. Let the squash cool, then remove and discard the seeds and stringy membranes. Scoop out enough squash flesh to measure 1 cup; reserve any remaining squash for another use. Leave the oven at 375° F.

Lightly spray 2 baking sheets with cooking spray. In a medium-size bowl stir together the flour, oats, baking soda, ginger, allspice and salt; set aside. In a large bowl, using an electric mixer, cream the margarine and sugar until thoroughly blended. Beat in the egg, then gradually beat in the squash and vanilla. Add the dry ingredients and beat for 5 to 10 seconds, or just until mixed, then stir in the apricots, currants and prunes. Drop the dough by rounded teaspoons onto the baking sheets and bake for 12 minutes, or until the cookies are golden at the edges. Transfer the cookies to racks to cool and repeat with the remaining dough.   Makes 96 cookies

CALORIES per cookie	23
69% Carbohydrate	4 g
7% Protein	.4 g
24% Fat	.6 g
CALCIUM	4 mg
IRON	.2 mg
SODIUM	17 mg

PROP CREDITS

Cover: tank top–Athletic Style, New York City, leotard, tights–Dance France, LTD., Santa Monica, Calif., shoes–Nautilus Athletic Footwear, Inc., Greenville, S. C., barbell, dumbbell–The Fitness Stop, Inc., New York City; page 6: shirt, shorts–Athletic Style, New York City; weight belt and location courtesy of Madison Avenue Muscle, Inc., New York City; page 24: unitard–Danskin, Inc., New York City, trunks–Marika, San Diego, Calif.; page 28: dumbbells, barbells, weights–Gemfitness, New York City, ankle weights–Triangle Health and Fitness Systems, Morrisville, N.C., mat–AMF American, Jefferson, Iowa, towel–Martex, New York City; pages 30-55: shirt, Naturalife, New York City; sweats–Russell Corporation, Alexander City, Ala.; sneakers–Nautilus Athletic Footwear, Inc., Greenville, S.C., barbell–Gemfitness, New York City, dumbbells–Triangle Health and Fitness Systems, Morrisville, N.C., mat–AMF American, Jefferson, Iowa, chair–Conran's, New York City, step stool–The Pottery Barn, New York City, sheet and towel–Martex, New York City, rug–ABC International Design Rugs, New York City; page 56: leotard, tights–Dance France, LTD., Santa Monica, Calif.; pages 60-79: leotard, tights–Dance France, LTD., Santa Monica, Calif., sneakers–Nautilus Athletic Footwear, Inc., Greenville, S.C., location courtesy of Ralph Anastasio, The Printing House Fitness Center, New York City; page 80: shirt, shorts–Athletic Style, New York City, sneakers–Avia, Alexandria, Va.; pages 84-123: shirt, shorts–Athletic Style, New York City, sneakers–Avia, Alexandria, Va., location courtesy of Mike Motta, Plus One Exercise Fitness Clinic, New York City; page 128: linen napkin–Ad Hoc Softwares, New York City; page 13: cheese grater courtesy of Francine Kass; page 131: plates–Sointu, New York City, glasses–Platypus, New York City, linen napkins and napkin ring–Ad Hoc Softwares, New York City, tile–Ceramique François, New York City; page 133: bowl, plate–Mood Indigo, New York City; page 134: plates, flatware–Sasaki, New York City, glasses–Frank McIntosh at Henry Bendel, New York City; page 138: plates–Daniel Levy Ceramic, New York City, wicker tray–The Pottery Barn, New York City; page 141: linens–Ad Hoc Softwares, New York City.

ACKNOWLEDGEMENTS

Our thanks to Michael D. Wolf, Ph.D., for his assistance

All cosmetics and grooming products supplied by Clinique Labs, Inc., New York City

Nutrition analysis provided by Hill Nutrition Associates, Fayetteville, N.Y.

Off-camera warm-up equipment: rowing machine supplied by Precor USA, Redmond, Wash.; Tunturi stationary bicycle supplied by Amerec Corp., Bellevue, Wash.

Washing machine and dryer supplied by White-Westinghouse, Columbus, Ohio

Index prepared by Ian Tucker

Production by Giga Communications

PHOTOGRAPHY CREDITS

Exercise photographs by Andrew Eccles; food photographs by Steven Mays, Rebus, Inc.

ILLUSTRATION CREDITS

Page 9, illustration: Brian Sisco; page 10, illustration: David Flaherty; page 13, illustration: Brian Sisco; page 14, illustration: David Flaherty; page 15, chart: Brian Sisco; pages 18, 19, illustration: David Flaherty; pages 22, 23, illustration: David Flaherty; page 59, illustration: David Flaherty; page 83, illustration: David Flaherty.

INDEX